# ALLERGIES & YOUR FAMILY

### Doris J. Rapp, M.D.
### F.A.A.A., F.A.A.P.

Clinical Assistant Professor of Pediatrics
at the State University of New York at Buffalo

**Sterling Publishing Co., Inc.   New York**
Distributed in the U.K. by Blandford Press

Library of Congress Cataloging in Publication Data

Rapp, Doris J
  Allergies and your family.

  Includes index.
  1. Allergy. 2. Pediatric allergy, 1. Title.
[DNLM: 1. Allergy and immunology—Popular works.
WD300 R221ab]
RC584.R368          616.97          79-93250
ISBN 0-8069-5558-9
ISBN 0-8069-5559-7 (lib. bdg.)
ISBN 0-8069-8878-9 (pbk.)

Sixth Printing, 1984

# Contents

# PART SIX

## *Circumstances Creating Potential Problems for Allergic Persons*

# PART SEVEN

## *Special Aids to Help Those with Allergies*

# Acknowledgments

It is extremely difficult to write a book autonomously. The following people, by suggestions and encouragement, helped to ease my qualms about the quality of the following pages.

Thelma Brock, M.D.; Winifred Mernan, M.D.; Merwyn Garrett, M.D.; George Kunz; Rita Smyth, Ed.D.; Dr. and Mrs. Daniel Fahey; Francis Ehret, M.D.; Anthony Runfola, M.D.; Pat Wilson; Phyllis Forton; Joanne Brown, R.N.; and Dr. C. Guzzetta.

There is little in this book that is truly original. It is basically my individual distillation of the medical knowledge that many capable allergists have gradually accrued over the years. The writings and attitude of Jerome Glaser, in particular, of Harry L. Mueller and Susan Dees have been major influences helping to mold my own personal philosophy and methods concerning the practice of allergy.

# Foreword

This book was written to help you understand more about your allergies and the allergies of other members of your family, especially your children. I have specifically tried to explain what *you* can do to help determine what is causing an allergy. I describe how you might be able to delay or prevent the development of an allergy.

This book may reveal that you have allergies of which you weren't even aware. It may suggest additional avenues of self-help for those patients already receiving allergy treatment.

The basic principles guiding the treatment of allergies are the same whether you are two years old or fifty. It does not matter whether the allergies affect the nose, chest, eyes, ears, digestion, disposition or nervous system—the methods used to relieve patients are the same. Medicines are often helpful. In addition, many children and about half of the adults who have allergies are helped by altering conditions within their home, by changing what they eat, by taking allergy-extract injection treatments or avoiding chemicals or pollutants.

Medicines used to relieve allergies are usually effective, but as soon as the medicine is not taken, the problem recurs. If you want to eliminate allergies more permanently, attempts must be made to determine what is causing the symptoms. If a nail in your shoe is causing a sore on your foot, it helps to put medicine on the sore, but the real solution to the problem is to remove the nail. This book is written to help you find the "nails" causing your allergy problems.

Let's talk about how you can use this book most effectively. Read Chapter 1 first. It answers the general questions you may have wondered about and possibly may help you decide if you have an allergy. Next, read the chapters in the book which specifically discuss your kind of allergy. For example, if you have a nose or eye allergy, read Chapter 2. If you cough or wheeze, read Chapter 3. Next, you must know something about the types of medicines or drugs used to treat allergies; therefore, read Chapter 12. This chapter helps to explain exactly what these medicines are supposed to do, and, equally important, what they are *not* supposed to do.

At this point, you should try to decide if and how your allergies might be helped. If your allergies are worse when you are outdoors, especially during the warmer months, it often indicates that airborne pollen or mold spores (see pages 12 and 13) are causing your difficulties. This type of allergy causes symptoms at almost the same time each year for a few days or weeks. If your seasonal allergies interfere with normal activity, either work or play, your physician can recommend medicines to help decrease your symptoms. You might also need to see a physician who has special training in allergy so that you can have allergy skin tests (Chapter 10) and receive allergy-extract injection treatments (Chapter 11). During the time when symptoms are evident, it may help if your bedroom is especially well-cleaned so that as many allergenic items as possible can be eliminated (Pages 21-22 and Chapter 8). An air-purifier (page 125) or one of the new so-called HEPA filters might also be of benefit.

If your allergies occur all the time, every day, or on and off throughout the year, you might want to try the methods outlined in the following paragraphs. Sometimes these measures help in a few days, but if you're not significantly better after a few weeks, you need more help from an allergist. These measures aid mainly the type of allergy that aggravates or inconveniences a patient (*e.g.*, a constant stuffy nose or throat-clearing). If your allergies are incapacitating, you need personalized care from an allergist.

\*    \*    \*

If your allergy is worse when you are indoors and improves when you are on vacation, camping, in a hospital or visiting friends, the cause of your difficulty is probably inside your home. (Sometimes you may notice no difference, however, because the place you visit may contain the same allergenic item which is found in your home.) Allergies due to factors in your house may tend to improve in the warm months when the windows are open and get worse during the colder months or when you first get up each morning. See Chapter 8 and pages 282 to 288 for suggestions on what to do to make your home more "allergy-free." A room air-purifier is sometimes necessary for maximum improvement. This is especially true if you live in a very dusty old home, have pets, or simply want to do everything you can to help delay or decrease the possibility of developing seasonal pollen allergies. If odors bother you, chemical sensitivities may be a problem.

\*    \*    \*

If your allergies began in *infancy,* a food is very often the cause of the problem. This is true even if you are 40 years old, *provided* the symptoms *began* when you were a baby. It is possible, however, to develop a food allergy at any age. Food allergies tend to persist no matter where you live or travel.

A runny nose, indigestion, coughing or wheezing, eczema, headaches, muscle aches and even some hyperactivity, irritability, bladder problems and fluid retention can be due to a food. Different types of diets are called for depending upon whether the problems occur intermittently or continuously. If you don't have any idea which food might be at fault, try the *Multiple Elimination Diet* described on pages 147 to 165. This eliminates some of the major foods which are often the cause of food allergies.

In summary, if you are not better after changing your household conditions for two weeks, try the diet for one-two weeks and see if that helps. If you think your problem is more apt to be a food allergy, try the diet first. If you are in a hurry, try both the household changes and the diet at the same time. In about two to four weeks you should be able to tell if these measures have relieved your symptoms. If you are not better, you've probably done as much as you can on your own. You will need advice from an allergist.

\* \* \*

The measures I've suggested won't help everyone to the same degree. Sometimes no matter how hard you or even your doctor tries, the cause of your allergy can't be determined. The important point, however, is that you try to figure it out. The information you discover may provide your doctor with the answers he needs so that he can help you to a greater degree.

In this book I've tried to stress what *you* can do to help yourself. Any advice, however, which you follow should be discussed first with your own physician or allergist. Only your physician knows your personal health problems. He can guide you while you try to carry out the general suggestions which have been outlined, and he can adapt your allergy care to your specific needs.

Doris J. Rapp M.D
F.A.A.A., F.A.A.P.

# PART ONE

# Basic information

This section includes candid practical answers to the general questions which allergic patients or parents of allergic children often ask. It explains the different symptoms which can be due to an allergy and what is commonly thought to cause this type of medical problem. It discusses various factors such as heredity, age when allergies begin, outgrowing the problem, the effect of weather, and why allergies are in some ways easy and in other ways difficult to treat. It helps to explain what you might do to help yourself and when you might need the help of an allergist. It tells approximately what allergy treatment will cost and where such care can be obtained.

# CHAPTER 1

# *General questions most parents ask*

**What is an allergy?**

An allergy is an abnormal response to a food, drug, or something in our environment which usually does not cause symptoms in most people. We do not know exactly why some persons develop an abnormal response, for example, to ragweed pollen or to fish, while others do not. At least ten to 20 per cent of the population have some manifestation of allergy at some time in their lives. Allergies can begin at any age. Substances which cause allergies are called allergens or antigens.

**Are allergies hereditary?**

Allergies are not really hereditary in that a father who has asthma or wheezing caused by grass pollen does not necessarily have children who wheeze because of exposure to grass. Allergies to specific substances, such as grass, are not inherited. Some families do, however, tend to have chest allergies (asthma), while others may have mainly hay fever. Identical twins, for example, don't always both develop allergies. The genetic inclination to develop allergies, however, does tend to be evident in certain families. If both parents have severe allergies, their children are more apt to have many symptoms of allergies.

Children with such strong hereditary tendencies may not only develop allergic symptoms in infancy, but these symptoms may also be more severe and varied. Such an infant could have colic, eczema, asthma and nasal allergies, all before the age of one year. Of course this tendency to develop allergies will be much less if only one distant relative has this problem. If a youngster's only allergic relative is an asthmatic great-grandfather, this child may never manifest allergies, or he might develop mild hay fever in middle age. The symptoms in this type of person would often tend to be less severe and have their onset later in life.

## What areas of the body are affected by allergies?

The part of the body which is affected by an allergy is called a shock organ. The common ones are the skin, nose, eyes, chest, intestines, or ears. A single substance that causes allergies can affect one or many different areas of a child's body. For example, milk can cause eczema and abdominal pain, while another allergenic substance such as ragweed pollen can cause asthma and hay fever in the same child.

1. Skin allergies are usually called:

eczema or atopic dermatitis (often a rash in the creases of the arms or legs) (See Chapter 4.)
contact dermatitis (tiny, itchy blisters in the skin)
urticaria or hives (swellings similar to mosquito bites, swollen lips, or swollen eyes). (See Chapter 6.)

2. Nose allergies are characterized by watery, nasal mucous secretions, stuffiness, sniffing, snorting, sneezing several times in a row, throat-clearing, an itchy or wiggly nose, or rubbing the nose upward. (See Chapter 2.)

3. Eye allergies usually affect both eyes, and are manifested by watery secretions, itchiness, and redness due to rubbing. (See Chapter 2.)

4. Chest allergies are associated with a repeated cough which does not respond to the "common" medicines. If the cough is hoarse or barky it often indicates infection and not allergy. Asthma is one cause of wheezing and this means that, as the child breathes out, the air whistles in his chest. If the asthma is very severe, there is also a squeak as he breathes in. (See Chapter 3.)

5. Gastrointestinal allergies can cause a bellyache, nausea, abdominal discomfort, diarrhea, constipation, an excess of mucus or gas, or halitosis.

6. Ear allergies commonly cause intermittent hearing loss or recurrent ear problems because of fluid behind the eardrum. (See Chapter 2.)

7. Less common allergies include headaches, a geographic tongue (that is, one having a patchy or spotty appearance), disposition change, hyperactivity, fatigue, muscle aches, arthritis, joint swelling, recurrent cold sores (see p. 177), seasonal bladder problems, vaginal irritations, bed-wetting, heart, blood vessel and kidney problems.

## What causes an allergy?

An allergy can be caused by a multitude of substances. See pages 276 and 277.

1. "Winter" or year-round allergies, whether daily or intermittent, are mainly caused by:

house dust
furniture stuffing such as kapok, cotton, hair, rubber or polyurethane
foods (eaten or smelled)
wool, fur, or feathers (pets)
mold spores and algae
insect debris
pleasant-smelling substances (such as deodorizing aerosols, perfumes, lotions, bubble bath, powders, scented facial or toilet tissue). (See p. 266 under section on "Orris Root.")
chemical odors (gas, gasoline, plastic, Lysol, oil, etc.).

At any time certain nonspecific irritants can trigger allergic symptoms. Examples would be dirt, tobacco smoke, burning leaves or rubbish, sawdust, exhaust fumes, or chemicals and odors in the air.

2. "Spring" allergies[1] are mainly caused by:

mold or other contaminants on grass after the snow melts: late March
various tree pollens: very late March through June
early grass pollens: early to mid-May through early July.
Many trees develop tiny flowers, usually just before the leaves unfold, and the pollen is abundant in the air for a week or two from each type of tree. When the flowers have dropped off, there can be no pollen and so the tree no longer causes allergies.
In the Northeast, trees pollinate roughly in this order:
silver maple: very late March or early April
elm: April
poplar: late April and early May
birch, ash, oak, and other maples: late April or May.
Fruit trees, chestnut, Norway maple, locust, and willow are not wind- but insect-pollinated and supposedly do not cause allergies. (Use these, therefore, to landscape your property if your child has allergies.)

3. "Summer" allergies[1] are mainly caused by:

various grass pollens: mid-May to early July
various mold spores: mid-July to first frost or October.
The various types of grass pollinate in a definite sequence starting with the early lawn grass in mid-May, followed by June and orchard grass, and ending with red top, timothy and rye in early July.
Mold spores are similar to the mold seen on moldy bread, but the types which cause allergies are found in the air during the summer. They can

[1] These times refer only to northeastern U.S. Pollination will vary within the area or region where the patient lives; for more complete breakdown, see Appendix, pp. 278 to 281.

also be found on fallen leaves and on other vegetation in the late fall. Some damp homes are contaminated with molds throughout the year or during humid periods.

Some common mold spore types are *Alternaria, Hormodendrum, Aspergillus, Fusarium, Monilia,* or *Penicillium.* (A sensitivity to the latter is unrelated to a sensitivity to the antibiotic penicillin.)

4. "Late summer" allergies[1] are mainly caused by:

various mold spores (see above): mid-July through first frost
various weed pollens: from mid-August to first frost.
Ragweed is the most common pollen, but there are many other pollens, such as burweed marsh elder, cocklebur, lamb's-quarters, pigweed and wormwood. All of these can contribute to a child's symptoms. Ragweed is a minor problem in parts of northern Michigan and Maine. (Vacation or live in these areas if ragweed is a major problem.)

## What is pollen?

Pollen is a common allergen or antigen. It is an airborne, spermlike substance. Plants which cause allergies are usually drab, green and inconspicuous—not pretty colored flowers. In the eastern United States,[1] the allergies noted in June are not caused by brightly colored roses (often called "rose fever") but are from grasses. Allergies in the late summer (mid-August to the first frost) are not caused by the bright yellow goldenrod but by ragweed or other inconspicuous weeds. Pollen of the latter type can travel for many miles since it is very light, plentiful, buoyant and spread by the wind. Pollen granules are usually yellow in color and only 10 to 30 microns[2] in size; most can only be identified microscopically. Pollination occurs mainly between 4 and 8 A.M. If you shake a plant at the time that it is pollinating, you can often see a cloud of yellow dust which consists of pollen. You can also tell if a plant is pollinating by putting it gently on a piece of white paper. After a few hours the yellow pollen will be obvious.

## Can brightly colored flowers cause allergies?

Yes, although in their natural setting they do not. Bright flowers have only a small amount of pollen which is very sticky and heavy. The bright flowers attract bees. Pollen sticks to the body of the bee, and is spread from plant to plant as the bee flits about. This type of pollen causes difficulty only if a bouquet is brought into a room or if, for example, a child repeatedly picks and sniffs dandelions.

---

[1] See Appendix, pp. 278 to 281, for pollination times in each state.
[2] A micron ($\mu$) is one-thousandth part of a millimeter. There are approximately 25 millimeters to one inch.

Dried flowers are often contaminated with molds or sprayed with paints or chemicals, all of which can cause allergic symptoms. Cocoons and dried plants such as teasel would be typical examples. Wild carrot, or Queen Anne's lace, in particular, is covered with molds in the fall.

Patients allergic to ragweed often have symptoms from exposure to chrysanthemums or zinnias. These plants have pollen which is possibly similar to ragweed pollen. Close contact is usually necessary before symptoms are noticed.

### Can you move away from pollen?

Not really. Any area which has green foliage has pollen. In the South, especially in certain parts of Florida or Texas, molds are a special problem. In the Midwest, at certain times the pollen concentration in the air is amazingly high compared to that of the East Coast. A child may be fine after a move to the West Coast, but often only until the western ragweed sensitivity replaces the eastern ragweed problem.

Parents who get upset because there are fields near their home which may expose their child to undue amounts of pollen are not being realistic. Pollens blow for miles and, although it is certainly better not to live in the center of fields, persons in heavily populated urban areas also have pollen problems. Your child could, however, have worse maple-tree allergies if one is directly outside his bedroom window. But the maples which are blocks and blocks away from your home can also contribute to his allergic problems.

### Can a substance cause allergies at one time and not at another?

Yes. A child can be allergic to ragweed, but have no difficulty when the concentration of ragweed pollen in the air (ragweed count)[1] is low. Symptoms of hay fever might be noted when the count is moderate and symptoms of both hay fever and asthma may occur when the count is very high. The amount of the substance needed to cause symptoms in an individual is called his allergic threshold.

Most allergic children are sensitive to more than one substance. It is not unusual for one child to be sensitive to many different things. Whether a child has symptoms or not at any particular time would depend upon how much and how many of these substances were in the child's contact or surroundings at a particular time. A massive exposure

---

[1] A ragweed "count" is a number often published daily during the fall season in many newspapers to give a rough indication of the amount of ragweed pollen in the air. Low counts in New York State would possibly be under 25, high ones over 75 particles per square centimeter.

to only one of them could cause symptoms, or a little exposure to many of the allergenic substances, all at once, could cause difficulty. Some children, for example, have no difficulty when exposed to their dog, except when their dog is shedding. Some children who cannot eat cantaloupe or melon during the ragweed season can do so at other times of the year.

### Can you determine the cause of your child's allergies without the help of an allergist?

Yes. Sometimes a mother, for example, can determine the cause better than the physician because she can observe her child constantly. The allergy specialist can sometimes only give suggestions concerning probable factors based on his experience and knowledge. Remember, however, that the obvious is not always the cause of the problem. You can drink rye and water, gin and water, and vodka and water. It is not the water causing the obvious effect. If a child is allergic to orange, difficulty can be noted with a fresh orange, an orange popsicle, an orange-flavored beverage, orange-flavored gelatin and orange-flavored medicine. Unless a parent watches very carefully, it could easily be missed that the orange dye or flavoring was at fault. It requires a detective-like imagination to deduce the causes of allergies. Parents and children can often determine exactly what causes an episode of asthma or hay fever by thinking about what the child was doing, where he played and what he touched, ate or smelled just prior to the attack. Symptoms may occur in minutes or several hours later.

### What are some indications that your child needs an allergist?

If symptoms interfere with normal activities, such as school attendance or play activity, then the allergies should be evaluated professionally. Many children under two years of age wheeze with each infection but, if this only happens once or twice, an allergist may not be needed. If, however, the wheezing is a recurrent problem or if the nasal allergic symptoms are severe, then an allergist should be seen. Allergies can make some children prone to recurrent colds or infections, ear or hearing problems and nosebleeds. At times these also should be evaluated by an allergist. An allergist's recommendations may prevent future allergies.

### Who is an allergist?

Most qualified allergists have successfully completed their specialty requirements, including board examinations in pediatrics (specialists for children) or internal medicine (specialists for adults), or have separate board certification in allergy. This training almost always indicates that the allergist is truly a specialist in the detection and treatment of allergic problems. Many equally interested and competent physicians practicing allergy are very capable although they may not necessarily be certified. There are, of course, marked individual differences among physicians. A doctor's success in treating an allergy depends not only upon his training and background knowledge but also upon his thoroughness, insight, and personality.

**How can you determine who is a qualified allergist in your area?**
Contact the County Medical Society and ask them for names of the nearest board-certified allergists.

**What does an allergist do?**
An allergist must first determine whether a child's symptoms are truly caused by allergies. If the diagnosis is correct, then the physician must decide if symptoms are serious enough to warrant treatment or further investigation. At times, only prophylactic advice is necessary to help prevent future serious allergic symptoms.

The specialist will prescribe medications in an effort to prevent or control the symptoms which your child has. These, however, will help only temporarily. If a child has a nail in his shoe causing a sore on his foot, the most effective treatment is not to put an ointment on the sore, but rather to pull out the nail. Giving medicine to treat hay fever or an asthmatic episode is like putting ointment on the sore. It will not solve the basic, underlying problem. The major concern of an allergist is to "pull out the nail" or to determine exactly what is causing allergic symptoms in the child. At times, the cause is obvious and simple avoidance of an offending substance will eliminate the problem so that drugs are not needed.

Changes in a child's surroundings or diet can at times completely stop his symptoms. If, however, the cause of an allergy is unknown, or if it is difficult or impossible to avoid an offending substance, allergy skin testing may have to be done. These tests help to pinpoint the cause of an allergy and determine the degree of the sensitivity. From these skin-test reactions and a knowledge of exactly when a child has symptoms, the allergist frequently prepares one or more extract medicines. These are a combination of various substances to which a child is sensitive as determined by skin testing and for which the allergist feels a child should and can be treated. Injection treatments of these extract medicines are believed to cause a child to form protection inside his body so that future exposure to these substances, which previously precipitated symptoms, will be less of a problem. The problems of most allergic children are treated by a combination of changing certain aspects of a child's home, diet, or by allergy-injection treatments.

### Can a child's condition improve if parents do nothing other than make their home "allergy-free?"

This should always be the first suggestion carried out by parents because it is often the simplest, least expensive and most rewarding. A stuffed toy, dusty furnace or family cat could be the major or sole cause of the child's problem; improvement following its removal is often dramatic. This form of treatment, however, would be inadequate if a child had significant symptoms during a pollen season. In some children, however, if the symptoms were *mild* when pollens and mold spores were in the air, it might be possible, by installing an air-purifier (see pp. 125–128) in the bedroom, to diminish symptoms to such a degree that injection treatments could be delayed or possibly even avoided.

### Can a child's allergies subside if dietary studies only are carried out?

This again is very possible in some children. This would be especially true for a child whose symptoms date back to early infancy or if his problem were a daily one. The usual foods causing allergies and methods of testing for these are detailed in Chapter 9. In some patients elimination of foods may diminish the child's problem to such a degree that further investigation of the allergies is not necessary. For example, it is possible for a child to have a constantly stuffy or runny nose, and by eliminating milk from this child's diet, complete improvement will be seen. In other children the nasal problem may subside to such a degree that only slight morning stuffiness persists. For a minimal problem such as this, lasting perhaps five minutes in the morning, complete skin testing and years of treatment with extract may be more trouble than they are worth.

### Can a child improve if treated only with allergy-extract injections?

It certainly might be possible for some children to improve if they were only to receive injection treatments, without consideration of the home conditions, foods or other possible factors causing the allergies. There is little doubt, however, that the more comprehensively and vigorously the problem is attacked, the sooner and more completely a child will improve. The more cooperation and genuine interest the

EXAMPLES OF ALLERGY THRESHOLDS

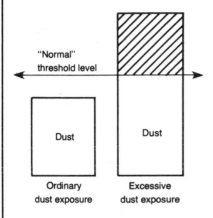

This shaded area shows that the excess dust above the threshold causes symptoms.

This shows how a child who is allergic to dust has no symptoms when the total dust exposure is below the child's threshold for symptoms.

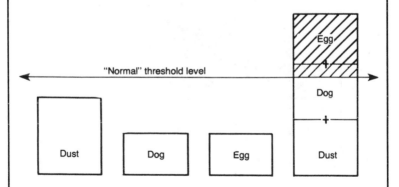

This shows how a child who is allergic to dust, dog and egg has no symptoms when exposed to each separately in a small or less-than-the-threshold level. If, however, the combined exposure exceeds the threshold level, then symptoms occur.

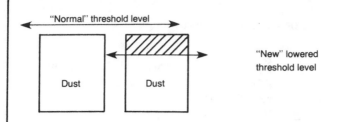

This shows that a certain amount of dust does not cause symptoms of allergy at a time when the threshold is "normal," while it will at a time when the threshold is lowered. The usual causes of a lower-than-normal threshold are infection, chilling, fatigue, exercise or an emotional stress.

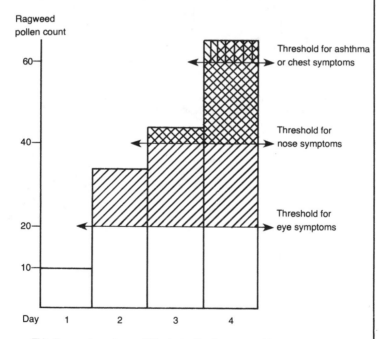

This diagram shows how a child who is allergic to ragweed has no symptoms when the ragweed count is below 20, has eye symptoms when it is above 20, eye and nose symptoms when it is above 40, and eye, nose, and chest (asthma) symptoms when the count is over 60.

parents, physician and the patient himself show, the sooner an allergic youngster will respond to treatment. It is foolish to receive injections for feathers if all you need to do is to remove your feather pillow.

### Do all children with allergies need extract-injection treatments?

No. If the symptoms are mild and don't happen very often, a child may not need any medicine. If the symptoms can be controlled by a little medicine, such as an occasional antihistamine, it is not necessary to see an allergist. Family physicians refer children to allergists when the symptoms are severe enough to warrant additional evaluation or study. This is usually required if uncontrollable nasal symptoms or repeated wheezing are noted. Your allergist will then decide if extract-injection treatments are essential. Many infants will have their allergic symptoms subside after their environment is altered or their diet changed. This also is true of some older children and adults. An old feather pillow, comforter or mattress could be the sole cause of a child's problem, but usually it is more complicated. Older children are more likely to be allergic to many substances or odors.

### What should parents do if their child responds poorly to the "usual" allergy treatment and recommendations?

The first step would be to review the list of original recommendations which your allergist gave you and honestly check to see if you carried them out. Most patients are helped by making the home relatively allergy-free, checking for food allergies and receiving the extract-injection treatments. If a child is not helped by these measures, after a reasonable period of time—*i.e.,* at least six months and at most two years—then some different and possibly expensive studies would be indicated. Discuss the entire problem with your allergist and see what his present suggestions are. These are a few factors which parents, in particular, should consider if their youngster is doing poorly:

1. Has the bedroom gradually become less and less allergy-free with time? Is it dusty or cluttered?

2. Has the bedroom's location or the contents of the room been changed? Are the mattress and box springs *completely* encased? Are the encasings torn? Is the bedroom register or radiator covered? Have vaporizers made the wallpaper moldy? Could your child be allergic to the plastic mattress cover or synthetic mattress or blankets?

3. Have you acquired any new sources of allergy, such as a furry pet, a carpet or stuffed furniture?

4. Have you moved? Your new home may be a problem. Insulation material, new, odorous carpets or curtains are suspect.

5. Have you changed your heating system in any way or remodeled or refinished your home? Is the furnace filter changed monthly? Is the vacuum cleaner functioning properly? Have you added air-conditioning? Is the electronic air-purifier working properly? Is it cleaned at least monthly?

6. Is the basement or house damper than usual? Was there a flood in the cellar? Is the dehumidifier working?

7. Does anyone in your family have any new hobbies? Odors of model airplanes and art supplies can cause symptoms.

8. Has your child started to eat even a little bit of the food which contributed to his previous symptoms?

9. Were the original dietary trials really carried out exactly as the physician recommended? Interpretation is sometimes difficult because of an infection or pollen season occurring during the dietary study.

10. Have you kept detailed records of exactly when your child has symptoms? What did he eat, touch or smell prior to the onset of symptoms?

11. Is your child worse or better the week before and after the extract-injection treatment?

12. Was your child's extract dosage decreased and not subsequently reraised because of the administration of fresh medicine or because he was overdue for a treatment?

13. Does your child repeatedly cough up green or yellow mucus which might indicate a chronic, low-grade sinus or lung infection?

The above applies equally to patients who have never responded favorably to treatment and to the rare child who does well and then suddenly seems to be worse again.


### Why are allergies difficult to treat?

Basically this is so because an allergy is not like an infection such as a sore throat. A child is not simply examined and given a medicine which solves the problem in a few days. It is much more complicated. Allergies usually recur until the causes of the difficulty are eliminated or the child is sufficiently treated for them. It is possible that a mother may have to drastically change parts of her home, her method of cooking and her child's diet. Her child may have to be skin tested and receive allergy-injection treatments for years. It means that records must be kept and she and her child's physician must be patient and cooperative, not for days or weeks, but for years. This is not easy, but it is the way that many children who have allergies are helped.

### If the help of an allergist is not available, how can parents determine and eliminate their child's allergies?

If a child does not have seasonal pollen symptoms, it is certainly possible for parents to solve their child's allergic problems. This is especially true if the symptoms occur daily or intermittently *throughout* the year.

The first recommendation made by many allergists is to make your home, and in particular your child's bedroom, allergy-free. Chapter 8 details exactly how this can be done. Try it for two weeks and see if your child is not better. Many times dramatic improvement can be seen overnight or in just a day or two. If the child's problems are not helped or if the symptoms are only partially diminished, the next step would be for you to carry out dietary studies.

In Chapter 9, a number of diets with menus and recipes are outlined which omit some of the major foods most apt to cause allergies. Place your youngster on a diet and see if there is any improvement in one week. If there is, re-add, *in excess,* one at a time, the foods which were omitted. If the symptoms return, one or more of the foods which was re-added caused the difficulty; Chapter 9 tells you exactly how to find the offending foods. If you re-add each food in excess and your child is not better or worse, it is doubtful that *these* foods are a factor.

The above measures may help many children; those for whom there is still a problem need to see an allergist for more elaborate home study, dietary trials, and possible skin testing and treatment.

### Who should accompany a child to the allergist's office?

If at all possible, both parents should be with their child during the first visit to give the allergist the vital information and details required to help him make necessary decisions concerning their child's allergies. Parents often see different aspects of their child's illness and, as they present their personal interpretation, the physician can more completely and accurately analyze the problems. If only one parent can accompany the child, it should be the one who knows most about the child. Usually the mother has more information, although this is not always true.

If a friend or relative is sent with a child, the visit to the allergist will be of much less value. The physician can do a thorough physical examination, but in the field of allergy a detailed, thorough history is *so vital* that few major decisions can be made without it.

### Can a child be too young to have his allergies treated?

No. The sooner treatment is given, the better. However, a child should not be rushed to an allergist for the first bout of hay fever or asthma. If the problem becomes more frequent and more severe, regardless of the child's age, check with your physician about seeing an allergist. Very young children or infants are often remarkably easy to treat and require few skin tests or extract-injection treatments, sometimes none at all. The allergist would have to decide exactly how to treat each individual youngster whom he sees.

**Should your child be bathed before the initial visit to the allergist?**

By all means, bathe every child about to see a physician for the first time. Even patients with eczema should have a bath before seeing a doctor. The only exception should be an initial visit of an emergency nature.

Many parents are hesitant to bathe their youngster because he is ill. They are fearful that this could cause chilling. Such reluctance is unwarranted. Hospitalized patients are usually bathed daily and ill children at home can certainly be bathed in a warm bathroom, immediately dressed in warm pajamas, and placed in a heated bedroom.

**What sort of record-keeping will help your allergist?**

Keep a *simplified* calendar of exactly when your child has symptoms, what they are, and when you give your child medicine. With this information your allergist is best able to help your child. This may require a little time and thought, but such information can at times decrease a child's need for injection treatments by months or years.

You might use something like this:

| *Symptoms or Problems* | *Severity of Problems* |
|---|---|
| W–wheeze or asthma | + is slight |
| N–nose | +++ is severe |
| C–cough | ++ is anything in between |
| S–skin trouble or eczema | |
| I–infection | |
| H–hives | |
| E–eye | |
| Ea–ear | |

× means times medicine was taken, *i.e.*, 3× means 3 times that month

Example:

### AN ENTIRE YEAR'S RECORD

|  | Jan. | Feb. | Mar. | Apr. | May | June |
|---|---|---|---|---|---|---|
|  | N+ | N+<br>W++<br>I++ | H+ | W++<br>N+++<br>E+ | I++<br>N++ | W+ |
| Medicines for nose (eyes or skin): | none | 2× | 5× | 40× | 10× |  |
| Medicines for chest: | none | 10× |  | 30× |  | 1× |
| Miscellaneous factors: |  | anti-biotic | cat contact |  | anti-biotic |  |

|  | July | Aug. | Sept. | Oct. | Nov. | Dec. |
|---|---|---|---|---|---|---|
|  | ok | W++<br>N++ | W++<br>N+++<br>E++ | S+<br>W+ | S+++<br>N++ |  |
| Medicines for nose (eyes or skin): | none | 7× | 50× | 5× | 6× | 10× |
| Medicines for chest: | none | 8× | 10× |  | 2× |  |
| Miscellaneous factors: |  |  |  | no anti-biotic |  | ate choco-late |

If you want to make the record more exact, you can add the dates of the problem, the type of infection or its location, and anything special that might be related, such as exposure to a pet, to paint, being at camp or whatever you think may have caused the symptoms.

### Do allergies change with age?

They certainly do. Not only does the area of the body affected vary, but the substance causing allergy changes. For example, many extremely allergic infants initially have eczema, colic or intestinal problems caused mainly by foods. These problems are often outgrown by the age of two or three, only to be replaced with nasal allergies which are mainly caused by dust, molds, pets, pollens or scented substances. Often the mother interprets this phase as being a "constant mild cold" because her child has nasal symptoms but does not act sick. The next phase is excessive coughing for prolonged periods after infections. Exercise or exertion and emotional upsets, such as laughter or excitement, cause coughing. By about five years of age, wheezing is frequently noted, particularly with infections. Without proper allergy treatment it eventually can become an intermittent or daily problem which can occur for no apparent reason.

There are many exceptions to the above. Some infants telescope these symptoms so that they have eczema, hay fever and asthma all within their first year. Some lose their eczema when the nasal allergies begin and lose their nasal allergies when asthma begins. Others who are less fortunate keep acquiring new body locations for their allergies while retaining all their previous problems. Hyperactivity, fatigue, chronic headaches, muscle aches and intestinal or behavior problems can begin at any age. In some patients these are due to allergy. Proper and adequate allergy care at any point can help to eliminate your child's symptoms and measures can also be taken to prevent new allergic problems.

### Can a child "outgrow" his allergies?

Yes. Some appear to, but many do not. Some children have symptoms for a few weeks, months or years and then have little or no difficulty in the future. Studies in children have shown that if hay fever is treated only with antihistamines, about a third of the children will "outgrow" their problems in a few years; another third will continue with symptoms for many years and adjust to living with them. They use antihistamines when they need them and, unless their problem is very severe, they can play and carry on their usual activities. The remaining third develop an allergic cough or asthma, and these children should see an allergist. Children with hay fever who do not receive allergy treatment can become worse in adolescence.

Some allergic persons believe they have outgrown their allergy when actually they have merely been separated from its cause. An example would be a young man who enters the service or marries and finds that he no longer has allergic symptoms. The reason may be separation from the family pet, his favorite feather pillow, an old mattress, a musty cellar or some special food his mother frequently cooked for him. Some patients appear to be fine for years. Infection or stress often precede the recurrence of allergy—which can then last for years.

### What can happen if parents decide not to treat their child's asthma?

If the asthma is mild and infrequent, your child might be one of the fortunate youngsters who stops wheezing in time. Many youngsters, however, do not. The advantages of early treatment are as follows:

1. In general, the earlier asthma is treated, the easier it will be to determine the cause of the episodes and to control and prevent future attacks.

2. If the asthma is treated, your youngster can play and act like other children. It is very sad not to allow a child to play outside or in the cold because this causes asthma. Children are only children for a short time. If your child can be helped, it is not fair to deny him the simple joys of childhood, such as riding a bicycle or playing baseball.

3. It is true that it requires years of wheezing before we can measure the actual changes in the lungs caused by the asthma. But if the lungs are continually being damaged ever so slightly, the harmful effects gradually accumulate and, by the time the child becomes a middle-aged adult, it is possible to have an old-aged lung. An allergist can help to prevent or delay this.

4. Although children under the care of an allergist rarely die from asthma, do not feel that an untreated child cannot die. Without proper treatment, and sometimes even with the very best known treatment, it can happen.

**Why should a mother of an allergic child learn about allergies?**

The more a mother knows about allergies, the more she can help her child who has allergies and other children who could develop them. Asthma, for example, is at times a lifetime problem, even when the patient is under an allergist's care. A knowing mother can avoid bringing substances into her home which may cause allergies. She can be alert in recognizing early minor allergies in her other children and possibly eliminate offending substances immediately, so that future major problems do not arise.

**What role should fathers adopt in relation to their child's allergies?**

The father must assume the responsibility of learning as much as possible about his child's problem. The major difficulty which may arise for fathers is that many of them are working during the daytime and cannot accompany the mother and child on the initial visit to an allergist. At this visit an attempt is made to explain what needs to be done for the child and the reasons for doing it. When he misses this visit, the father often never really understands the necessity of making essential changes in his home or in his child's diet. Every attempt should be made to have both parents accompany the child during the first visit when the diagnosis and explanations are made. The last visit is also crucial because skin tests are interpreted and a future treatment plan is outlined. The intervening visits are usually for testing and the father's presence is less essential.

Caring for an allergic child is not always simple and mothers cannot and should not do it alone. There are times when the mother is not home in the evening, so the father must know which medicines to give and why. There are times when a mother has been up day and night for several days and, although the father is also fatigued, it helps greatly if he can occasionally give medicine at 3:00 A.M.

If either parent tends to be frightened and apprehensive when a child is wheezing, it is often most helpful if the other parent takes over. Whichever parent is the calmest should care for a frightened child. No parent wants to add to his child's problems, yet some people can't hide their emotions very well and this type of parent merely confirms the child's unwarranted fears. Have faith in your physician and the medicines which you have. Give the medicines and, if your child is not better, call your doctor.

### How are other children in the family of an allergic child affected?

Unfortunately, an allergic child can disrupt a normal family in many different ways. The type of home, heating, bedroom, meals and even landscaping may have to be altered. Sisters and brothers often resent the fact that they cannot own a pet or have a bedroom similar to their friends'. To the other children, it is better to make the physician rather than the allergic child responsible for these changes and restrictions.

Children who have severe allergies are often spoiled, in comparison with other children in the family. The ill child is often catered to, overprotected and even undisciplined because of his tendency to become ill. The other children may become resentful and jealous because of this. Even though the ill child is "always" going to the doctor and receiving injections, the siblings feel "left out." Sometimes they in turn develop behavior problems in their attempt to receive more attention.

Allergic children, even when only a few years old, can completely dominate an entire family. If their parents do not comply immediately with their wishes, they state that they will wheeze and, much to the parents' dismay, proceed to do exactly that. It does not require much conditioning before parents are afraid to say no, to set limits or to use their mature judgment.

The easiest method of handling this problem is to treat the allergic child as much like the other children as possible. Give rewards and punishment equally when they are due. The only exception is that medicine to prevent wheezing should be given to an asthmatic child about 20 minutes before any reprimand.

### When will symptoms appear if a child is exposed to something to which he is allergic?

It varies, among other things, with the degree of sensitivity. If a child is extremely allergic, a mere smell of the substance that causes difficulty is all that is needed for immediate symptoms to appear. If a child is less sensitive, it may require actual contact and might take a few minutes to an hour or two. If the allergy is less pronounced, it might be 24 hours, or even require a gradual build-up of the substance within the body over a week or so, before symptoms are noted. The substances which cause symptoms in a few hours or later are the most difficult to determine. The better detectives you and your allergist are, the sooner you will ascertain the cause of an allergic child's problems. The form of the substance would also alter the time needed before an allergic reaction might be noted. For example, a child could be allergic to fish. If the allergic symptoms appeared as soon as the child started to eat the food, it would indicate that undigested fish protein caused the problem. If, however, your child has no difficulty until several hours after eating the food, it means that your child is probably allergic to the digested form of the fish protein.

### Can the development of allergies be prevented in a child who has never had allergies?

Yes. If the substances that most often cause allergic symptoms are avoided, the onset of manifestations of allergy can be prevented or at least delayed. Dust can be decreased by using an electrostatic precipitation unit and by careful and thorough cleaning. Parents can decrease pollens in their home by using this same unit (see pp. 125--128). Kapok, feathers, horsehair, wool, pets, fur and pleasant-smelling substances (or chemical odors) can be avoided. Foods which often cause allergies can be avoided in early infancy. Mold contamination can be diminished in homes by using dehumidifiers. Don't buy or use items which have strong chemical odors, *e.g.,* synthetic carpets, draperies, furniture, soft plastic, insulation or magic markers. Avoid air pollutants, such as cigarette smoke.

### If a child is very allergic to many things, how much exposure to a new, highly allergenic substance is necessary before it causes difficulty?

It would vary depending upon the degree of sensitivity of the allergic individual. For example, there is very little or no ragweed pollen in many areas of Europe and the British Isles, and this is a highly allergenic substance. (We do not know, incidentally, exactly why this substance tends to cause so many allergies.) If someone with severe allergies moves from Europe to the United States, symptoms often will be noted in about two to three years after exposure to two or three ragweed-pollen seasons. Children who are very allergic can manifest symptoms to this substance by the age of two or three but seldom before. Pets are also highly allergenic, but at times a potentially allergic child can have a cat for years without symptoms, while another allergic child might have difficulty in a few months or sooner.

### How can you help your child if there is a sudden emergency allergic problem?

This sort of problem could arise if your child accidentally ate nuts and was extremely allergic to them; it can sometimes happen after an allergy-extract injection treatment. (See Chapter 11.) If you have allergy medicines, immediately give an antihistamine (a medicine used for nose, eye or skin allergies) *and* an asthma medicine. If these medicines don't help, or if you have none, contact your physician or go to the nearest hospital. A common error made by parents is to treat a sudden allergic problem with only one of the above medicines. A child who suddenly develops hives, swollen eyes or sneezing can cough or wheeze later on, even if he has never wheezed previously. The reverse can also occur. Both medicines, therefore, should be given. A single correct dose of an antihistamine and asthma medicine is not harmful under ordinary circumstances. If a food is the cause of a symptom (asthma, hay fever, hives, hyperactivity), Alka-Seltzer, *in gold foil,* or 1/2 tsp. baking soda in water may help.

### If your child is very ill with an allergy, can you retain your present physician and also request an allergist to see your child?

Yes. Chances are your physician will suggest a referral to an allergist for treatment of your child's problem. If he does not, merely ask him for an allergy consultation.

### Can an allergy cause tension or fatigue?

It certainly can. This is often seen in children who have eczema, nasal allergies or asthma. If your child had an even, lovable nature prior to the onset of the allergies, it is certainly possible that his agreeable disposition and personality will return once the allergies have responded to treatment. If, however, the youngster has always been difficult and emotional, he may have some other medical problem which needs attention, or he could possibly have had a food allergy since early infancy.

There are other children, however, who do not have typical allergic symptoms. The major complaint concerning these youngsters is that they seem restless, irritable, emotional, tense, sullen, tired and lethargic. Vague complaints of aches, discomfort and frequent crying are common. An individual child may fluctuate from extreme sluggishness and fatigue, despite an apparently adequate amount of sleep, to being so overactive that he is impossible to restrain. At times the child's behavior is so extreme that parents are concerned that brain damage or a severe psychiatric problem is present. These youngsters, however, may have what has been called an allergic tension-fatigue syndrome. Although the most frequent cause of this problem is a food, such as food coloring, sugar, milk, chocolate, eggs or corn, it is also possible that other common allergenic substances can be at fault (pollens, dust, molds, perfume odors).

### Does weather affect allergies?

There is no doubt that many children are affected by changes in weather. A completely adequate explanation for this cannot be given. Children often wheeze at night because of a wide variety of factors. Substances in the child's bedroom are probably the major cause, but variations in temperature, the position while sleeping or nightly hormonal changes can also be contributing factors. Many children tend to wheeze late in the afternoon, shortly after sunset. This may be precipitated by a sudden decrease in temperature. Many children wheeze when they breathe very cold air during the winter. This can be diminished by warming the air before it reaches the lungs. A scarf over the mouth or breathing through the nose helps. Childhood allergies often are worse when the weather is damp or when the barometer falls, especially if there is an associated rapid decline in temperature. Windy days, especially when there is much pollen in the air, make pollen-sensitive children much worse. Air pollution is related to various weather conditions, and any condition conducive to keeping air contaminants near the ground, such as a heavy fog, could contribute to an allergic child's symptoms.

### Does tobacco or cigarette smoke cause allergy?

Tobacco can act as a respiratory irritant in anyone, but definite proof exists that allergic infants and children can wheeze and develop hay fever symptoms when exposed to this type of air pollution. Smoking in confined areas, such as in automobiles, is especially irritating to the allergic child. The odor on clothing or hair can cause symptoms.

### Can a child be allergic to human hair or dandruff?

This has been suggested but never completely substantiated. Children can develop sudden symptoms, such as hay fever, asthma or a flare-up of eczema, in the barber shop or beauty parlor, but it is difficult to state with certainty what the offending substance is. It could be due to any substance used on the hair, such as oils, tonics, sprays or scented powders, or to dust, pollen or chemicals in the air. Egg-sensitive patients could have symptoms if exposed to egg-containing shampoos.

### Which chores should allergic children avoid?

Until children have been treated for their allergies and have responded so that symptoms are not in evidence, they should not be asked to help with any dusty work. This would include dusting furniture, using a vacuum cleaner or cleaning out any dusty area like a garage, cellar, closet, or attic. A boy who has symptoms whenever he is near freshly-cut grass should not mow the lawn. Children allergic to weeds cannot help with the weeding or maintaining the garden. Older children cannot spray insecticides, inside or outside of the house. Patients who have eczema on their hands should not wash dishes or use strong detergent cleaning solutions. Boys who wheeze in the cold cannot shovel snow. Most children can set the table for meals, dry dishes or help to keep the house or their rooms generally tidy. Older girls can help with the ironing or some cooking. Boys can remove garbage. When children no longer show sensitivity to various allergens, they can assume a greater contribution to the maintenance of the home.

### Are there any cautions for allergic children when they marry?

Ideally, of course, an allergic person should avoid marrying another allergic person. This, however, is not practical. Married couples who have allergies or many allergic relatives should be careful when they start housekeeping to follow the many prophylactic recommendations made in this book related to their home.

### What are all the costs, obvious and hidden, related to allergy testing and treatment?

Many parents find that they have very large drug bills prior to the time that an allergist is seen, yet their child is "always ill." After seeing the allergist, they will find initially that they continue to have many bills to pay but, hopefully, their child's health will start to improve.

1. *Testing Costs*. The initial cost of allergy testing will vary greatly depending upon whether your child has symptoms year-round or for only a few weeks seasonally. If these occur throughout the year and your child has many forms of allergy such as hay fever, asthma and eczema, the testing will cost more than if the problem is hay fever occurring only two weeks of the year. The cost of allergy testing varies in different parts of the United States. There is an individual variation, too, among allergists' charges.

2. *Extract Costs*. In most patients, one or more extract medicines are prepared after skin testing. These again vary in cost, depending mainly upon the ingredients, which are relatively expensive. With each new bottle, a few (usually three, at least) additional extract-injection treatments are needed because the fresh medicine is stronger. This is essential for safety reasons. Most extracts usually expire after a period of 12 to 18 months and must be replaced.

3. *Allergy-Extract Treatment Costs*. A physician will charge to give your child an allergy-injection treatment. If you have already paid for the extract, the injection-treatment charge will be less, since the physician does not have to add the cost of the extract to his fee. You are not paying for the time it takes the physician or nurse to give the treatment, but for the doctor's expertise.

Initially, the allergy-injection treatments are usually given one, two or three times a week. After a period of several weeks or months, some children would be placed on a three- or four-week schedule and at that point medical costs start to decrease. Many children have also started to show definite improvement at this point, so the drug bills are also less.

4. *Allergy-Evaluation Visit Costs*. One other cost would be for subsequent detailed visits to the allergist who needs to evaluate your child's improvement. These may be needed initially every few months, and later on every year or two. At that time, your child's original and subsequent records would be studied, and an attempt made to suggest other ways of helping your child. The ideal aim of an allergist is not improvement but relief of your child's symptoms to such a degree that eventually the allergy-injection treatments may be discontinued. This is certainly not always possible, but every attempt should be made to accomplish this goal. Preferably both parents (or the most informed parent) should be present for this visit. Some parents feel these visits are unnecessary and costly. It is conceivable for a child to receive

treatments for many "extra" years because of mild yearly symptoms. Regular reevaluation visits could possibly have eliminated the symptoms to such a degree that treatments would not have been necessary for so long a period of time.

### Can allergy testing be carried out in "free" clinics?

Yes. Patients on welfare or Medicaid may obtain free care in most of the larger city hospitals.

Sometimes, however, it is possible for clinic testing or treatment to be more expensive than private medical care. If a family is not on welfare or Medicaid and if the medical care at a hospital clinic seems expensive, compare the charges at an allergist's private office. Merely call an allergist and inquire. Do the same at local hospital allergy clinics.

### How does clinic allergy care compare with a private physician's allergy care?

Many patients who attend allergy clinics respond favorably to treatment. Some common disadvantages of clinic care are:

1. Your child may not see the same physician for each visit year after year.

2. Clinic patients often have to wait longer in a crowded waiting room to see the doctor.

3. The time spent with the physician may be much less.

4. Your child may be seen by physicians still studying allergy under the supervision of an untrained allergist.

5. There is often less time for detailed explanation since there are more patients to see and fewer physicians to see them. (Please remember that most practicing physicians in clinics are not paid. They are often volunteering the services on their one free morning or afternoon during the week.)

6. It is more than possible that a child receiving care in a clinic may be part of a research study. The physician in the clinic, however, would explain this to a parent prior to making his child part of such a program. If your child is part of a study, it is often possible that part or all of his treatment is really not treatment. Some children receive injections of water or sugar pills. If your child is in such a research situation, be certain to find out as many details as possible.

### Should you let your child know the extent of his medical expenses?

No. It is surely not your child's fault that he has allergies. He needs love and understanding and has enough burden to carry without his parents' telling him, even jokingly, that they would like to "send him back and get a well one" or that he is "really not worth all the money he is costing the family." A surprisingly large number of parents repeatedly make statements of this type in front of their sick child.

### Is there a stigma associated with having allergies?

There certainly should not be, but some misinformed persons believe that asthma or a food or drug allergy should be concealed. This attitude is incorrect and possibly even dangerous. By facing the problem squarely and receiving proper medical care, the allergies may no longer present themselves.

Unfortunate situations or even crises, which are preventable, can be avoided if the school nurse, gym teacher or summer camp director are adequately informed about your child's medical history. Emergency drugs should always be available.

### Do vitamins help allergy?

There are unsubstantiated claims that they do. In some patients, high doses of Vitamin C and B-complex, in particular, $B_6$, pantothenic acid and niacinamide seem to be helpful. Water-soluble vitamins are usually safe in large doses. If a physician supervises the use of large doses for several months and there is no improvement, it is unlikely that vitamins will help. The exact influence of trace metals and minerals is also nebulous in relation to allergy.

Some vitamins actually cause allergy because of a sensitivity to food coloring, corn, yeast, sugar or some other ingredient.

### Do adopted children have more allergies than other children?

I know of no studies in this regard, but the observation made by other allergists and myself is that they do. There also appears to be an increased incidence of hyperactivity and behavior problems in adopted children. One must wonder if prenatal nutrition and medical care might be a factor.

# PART TWO

~

# Common types of allergies

This section includes detailed information about the more common types of allergies which affect the nose, eyes, ears, chest or skin.

Chapter 2 tells how you can tell a cold from a nose allergy and how to temporarily help eye allergies. It also includes a discussion of ear allergies which are sometimes associated with a nose allergy.

Chapter 3 tells how you might be able to determine what is causing a cough. Also discussed is asthma, in particular extrinsic asthma, which is the most common variety.

Chapters 4 and 6 discuss the causes and treatments of two common types of skin allergy.

Chapter 5 will be of interest to the parents of highly allergic newborns or parents of children who began to have allergy shortly after birth.

Chapter 7 deals with unsuspected possible allergic diseases.

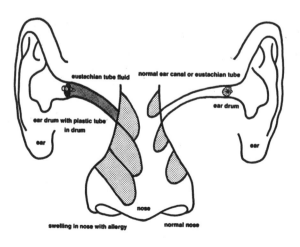

# CHAPTER 2

# Nose, eye, and ear allergies

## NOSE ALLERGIES

**What is hay fever?**

Hay fever includes nose and eye symptoms resulting from allergies. It affects up to ten per cent of the population. It has nothing to do with hay or fever. The usual medical term for this is allergic rhinitis ("rhin" refers to the nose and "itis" means inflammation) or, more correctly, allergic rhinorrhea ("orrhea" means flow). Patients can have seasonal allergic rhinitis, often called "seasonal pollinosis," or year-round symptoms called "perennial allergic rhinitis."

**What are hay fever signs and symptoms?**

Most children have one, or any combination, of the following:

1. Sneezing several times in a row, especially in the early morning.

2. Watery nasal mucous secretions.

3. Stuffiness (with or without watery mucous secretions), sniffling and snorting.

4. Mouth breathing.

5. Nose wiggling or wrinkling (like a rabbit) or mouth wiggling; some children massage the ends of their noses with their palms.

6. Nose rubbing or picking. The movement is rarely sideways but more frequently upward toward the forehead and this at times causes a characteristic allergic nose wrinkle across the bridge of the nose.

7. An itching in the roof of the mouth, ear canals or throat.

8. Throat-clearing.

9. Recurrent nosebleeds.

10. Inability to smell or taste.

11. Circles under the eyes, called "allergic shiners," or puffy eyes.

**How can you tell a cold from a nasal allergy?**

It is not always possible, because children can have both at the same time. Examination of the insides of the nostrils with a flashlight can often help in determining the cause of the nose problems.

|              | *Allergy*                            | *Infection*                  |
| ------------ | ------------------------------------ | ---------------------------- |
| Mucus is     | watery* and colorless; sometimes not evident | thick green, grey or yellow |
| Dried mucus  | none seen                            | many nose crusts             |
| Nose tissue  | more pale than lips                  | redder than lips             |

* Early in a viral infection the mucus may be watery, but it later becomes thick and colored.

If allergy and infection are present, a combination of the above will be seen.

Inside the curved part of the nostril, a mass of tissue can be seen called the "inferior nasal turbinate." If a patient has severe allergies, this tissue becomes very pale, frequently swells and enlarges so that it fills the inside of the nostril. The color changes from pink to bluish white.

Many infections are associated with fever or illness in other members of the family. Children with infection act ill, while those with allergies are more apt to be irritable.

**Does hay fever change a child's disposition?**

Yes. Hay fever patients are often irritable, listless, fussy, moody and touchy. Affected children tend to cry easily and not sleep as well as usual. Adults are often affected in a similar manner.

**At what times of the year do children have hay fever symptoms?**

Some children have symptoms only when pollens are in the air (pp. 278–281) or when they are exposed to cats or something to which they are sensitive. Others have symptoms all year, every day, particularly every morning.

**How are nose allergies treated?**

1. Whenever possible, the inhaled or eaten substance which is known to cause the allergy should be avoided. Electronic, portable air-filters are often helpful.

2. If the irritating substance cannot be avoided completely, it may

be possible to receive allergy-injection treatments for this substance.

3. Antihistamines (p. 207) often help to dry up mucus, to decrease swelling inside the nose and to diminish itching. If your child's nasal symptoms last only a few minutes after arising in the morning, there is no need for him to take antihistamines. These should be used only if the sneezing, stuffiness or watery mucus continues to be a problem for more than an hour, unless of course, the child is very uncomfortable.

4. Nose drops such as Neo-Synephrine, for which no prescription is needed, can be used. There is one strength for infants, another for children and a third for adults. (Some adult nose drops are unsafe for young children.) These drops help, but usually only temporarily. Many physicians do not recommend them. One reason is that some children tend to overuse them. Normally they should not be used more than two to three times a day or for more than two to three days. If they are used more often or for a longer period, some nose drops may irritate the inside of the nostrils and cause the membranes or tissue inside the nose to swell. The tendency to overuse nose drops occurs at this point and thus a vicious cycle begins.

Nose drops are considerably more effective if used in the following manner. Have your child lie so that his head is back and his nostrils face the ceiling. Put one or two drops in one nostril. (If you are using a spray, always have the nostrils facing the floor and spray once or twice.) Wait about five minutes, have your youngster blow his nose, and then repeat the procedure. Give the same amount in the same nostril. The first time you will shrink the tissue near the nose opening and the next time you will shrink the higher nasal membranes and clear the upper passageway. Repeat this same procedure for the other nostril.

Caution should be advised in the use of various medicated, Vaseline-like preparations which parents frequently place inside their youngster's nose to help to clear the nostrils. It is possible that these could irritate the inside of the nose in some children. Stop using them and see if your child breathes more easily or check with your physician.

5. There are masks which can be worn over the nose to prevent irritating substances from being breathed. This is an impractical means of solving the problem unless, for example, a child is allergic to dust and must clean a garage or basement or do a dusty chore in a small area.

6. Occasionally a cortisone nasal spray is used to treat nasal allergies, but this should never be used without a physician's close supervision.

7. Aspirin is often helpful in decreasing the effect of nasal allergies.

**What are common complications of hay fever?**

1. Bronchial asthma can occur. This is most often seen in patients who have severe hay fever symptoms. Some studies have shown that 30 to 60 per cent of children who have hay fever may subsequently develop asthma. Coughing in excess, in association with exercise or emotion, or shortness of breath is often a warning that chest allergies are imminent. It is possible, but fortunately would be uncommon, for a child who had only hay fever to develop asthma while receiving allergy-injection treatments. The treatments do not cause asthma. If it does occur, it is probably caused by an allergy to a new substance.

2. Recurrent infections are a frequent problem. Allergy causes the inside of the nose to swell, the membranes become less resistant to infection, the tissues become puffy and the blood supply is less than normal. It is not unusual to have germs or bacteria capable of causing infection in the nose and throat at any time. The allergic changes in the inside of the nose, namely swelling and paleness, tend to make some children more prone to infection. In children, infection tends to spread particularly to the ears and throat. In older children or adults, the sinuses are more apt to be affected, often causing headaches above or below the eyes. The chest can also be involved in either adults or children. Some physicians believe that if nose drops and antihistamines are used *immediately* at the first sign of infection, it helps to decrease the entrance of germs and tends to prevent or shorten infections.

3. Nasal polyps can occur. These are swellings inside the nose which look like the inside of a skinned grape and are usually very watery. Luckily, pre-adolescent children seldom have nasal polyps. This is fortunate because the condition is difficult to treat. At times, these polyps in adults are associated with chronic infection in the nose or with aspirin sensitivities (see p. 225). Patients with these problems always should be examined by a physician. Young children who have polyps could have cystic fibrosis.

4. Some children have recurrent nosebleeds. This is because the inside of the nose frequently swells, a condition which could stretch blood vessels to such a degree that the slightest trauma or rub could cause bleeding. The most common cause of nosebleeds, however, is not allergies but a delicate, superficial blood vessel which needs to be cauterized. In particular, the vessels may bleed in the area of the nose which separates the two halves. Another frequent cause is dried mucous crusts which lead to ''nose picking.''

5. Children who have severe nasal allergies for a long period of time often have a characteristic appearance to their face. From rubbing their nose upward they develop a horizontal crease or wrinkle across the top

of their nose. Because of the allergic swelling of the nose membranes, pressure within these tissues slows the proper drainage of blood vessels in the region of the eye, nose and sinuses. This causes what has been called "allergic shiners." These dark circles are very evident, especially when a child's nose has been very congested. The lower eyelid area often appears puffy. These children cannot breathe properly through their noses and as a result become mouth breathers or "allergic gapers." Prolonged use of the mouth rather than the nose for breathing tends to cause the mouth area of the face to become more prominent, while the nose area becomes less well developed by comparison. Dental deformities, in association with long, narrow palates, are not uncommon in children who have severe nasal allergies, and often require orthodontia.

### Can allergies cause a loss of smell?

Yes, this is possible. A loss of smell is sometimes noted in relation to food allergies or severe hay fever symptoms during a pollen season. Usually the sense of smell returns once the substance causing the allergy is avoided or if treatments are given to relieve the allergies (as with pollens).

### Are sinuses affected by allergy?

Yes, they are. The effect can be direct or indirect. Sinuses which are *directly* affected by allergies act as shock organs, in much the same manner as the lungs which are the shock organs for children who have asthma. The sinuses are air cavities located in the bones near the nose. The sinuses open into the nose through tiny passageways which allow air to pass into the sinuses and mucus to pass out of them. Mucus is normally formed by glands lining the sinuses and this mucus helps to keep the sinus cavities clean. If the membranes lining the sinuses are directly affected by allergy, they can swell and cause more than normal secretions to form. If the swelling is extreme, it can cause fluid to be trapped in the sinus cavity, and this creates a sinus headache. Such headaches are located above or below one or both eyes. If there are germs present in the mucus when it is trapped inside the cavities, this is called a sinus infection. This mucus is often green or yellow, and fever may or may not be evident.

Sinus problems are often *indirectly* caused by nasal allergies because the membranes lining the nose swell, blocking normal drainage from the sinus cavities. This in turn traps mucus or infection within the sinuses and causes headaches located in the bones surrounding the nose. Older children and many parents realize that they have sinus problems, but they are completely unaware of the fact that their basic difficulty is a nasal allergy. Morning stuffiness or sneezing several times in a row, an itchy nose and watery mucus all indicate nasal allergy and these can contribute to sinus problems. Large adenoids, deformities within the nose or diseased teeth are other common causes of sinus discomfort.

If a child's sinus problems are caused by allergies, the use of an antihistamine such as Tacaryl and nose drops will probably help temporarily. These drugs should shrink the allergically swollen tissues so that sinus drainage can occur. If infection is present, antibiotics would be indicated as directed by your physician. Heat applied to painful sinuses often helps to encourage drainage. The true solution to the problem, however, is to eliminate the cause of the allergic swelling inside the nose or sinuses, rather than to treat the effect.


## EYE ALLERGIES


**What are typical eye symptoms of allergy?**

Watery mucus, itching and redness caused by rubbing, generally affecting both eyes, are typical of allergies involving the eyes. One eye only could be affected if it were touched by something to which a child was sensitive. The usual causes—pollen, mold spores, scented substances, foods or dust—would affect both eyes. The diagnosis should be confirmed by a physician, since certain serious viral eye problems can cause similar symptoms.

**What causes yellow eye mucus?**

This would usually indicate infection. Children frequently have allergic eye itching and after vigorous rubbing introduce infection into their eyes.

**How can eye symptoms of allergy be relieved?**

1. Use Collyrium eye wash and an eye cup. Fill the eye cup with eye wash, at room temperature or very slightly warmed, and place it over the affected eye. Have your child blink several times and this will help to wash the offending substances from the front of the eyeball. (Having a child repeatedly open his eyes under the water while bathing in clear water would accomplish the same purpose.)

2. Put Collyrium eye drops with ephedrine or Estivan into the child's affected eyes. This medicine can be purchased inexpensively without a prescription and tends to diminish itching and irritation of the eyes.

Eye drops are easily applied if, with the child's head tipped backwards, a drop or two is put on the little pink spot in the inner corner of each eye. Do not touch the eye with the medicine dropper while doing this. Then pull down the lower eyelid, so that the drop of medicine will fall from the pink spot into the area between the eye and lowered eyelid. This will cause your child's eye to blink and it will spread the medicine over the front of the eye.

3. Have your child wear large and preferably curved sunglasses, since this will tend to act as a barrier and protect the eye from allergenic substances which might be in the air. This is particularly important if he is sitting near an open car window or riding a bicycle.

4. Give your child an antihistamine as directed by your physician. Some effective ones, such as Chlortrimeton and Tacaryl, can be purchased without prescription. Directions for use are on the bottle. This medicine should diminish the itching and possibly the swelling of the eye.

5. Try to keep your child's hands as clean as possible by washing them frequently with soap and water. This will reduce the possibility of introducing infection into the eyes when they are rubbed.

6. If these measures do not control eye symptoms adequately, stronger, more effective medicines can be obtained from your physician.

### Can the white part of the eye become very swollen from allergies?

Yes. At times the white part can bulge or swell to a very great degree. Your allergist should be contacted if this occurs. Measures described above should help temporarily but should not be carried out without your physician's approval.

### How dangerous is it for a child's eyes to swell completely shut?

This does not usually damage the eyes or the skin around the eyes, even though a youngster's face can be very distorted. An insect sting on the face, for example, can quickly cause the entire face to swell. Pollen blowing directly into the eyes, when a child is riding his bicycle against the wind, can cause the eyes to swell shut. Infection, unrelated to allergy, also can cause eyes to close from excessive swelling. A physician will therefore have to examine a child to determine the exact cause and treatment of this problem.

# EAR PROBLEMS

### Can recurrent problems in children's ears be caused by allergy?

Yes. Some cases of recurrent serous or secretory otitis are caused by allergy and respond to the usual type of allergy treatment. In addition, some of these children have typical nasal symptoms of allergy while others have only the ear problems.

### What causes chronic serous, or secretory, otitis?

This type of otitis is caused by the unnatural accumulation of fluid behind the eardrum within an area called the middle ear. The middle ear is a passageway which extends from the eardrum to the opening of the Eustachian (u-stay'-shun) tube, deep within the nasal passages. The middle ear, which is normally an airspace, becomes filled with fluid. If the Eustachian tube on the same side is not open, this in turn can cause a hearing loss. The Eustachian tubes normally open very frequently—for example, when swallowing occurs or during yawning or chewing. Air enters the middle ear when this occurs.

### What are the symptoms of chronic secretory otitis?

Parents or teachers may notice a mild to severe intermittent or daily hearing loss in these children. This is the usual cause for requesting that an ear specialist examine the child.

Some children have an associated feeling of fullness, blocked ears, crackling, popping or ringing in the ears. Some have pain or drainage. Fever is seldom evident. Both ears are usually affected, although one is often worse than the other. Some children surprisingly have no symptoms and the problem is not revealed until a child responds poorly during a routine hearing test in school. This type of otitis can begin in infancy but is most frequently evident at the age of three to ten years.

### Which methods of therapy help children who have fluid in the middle ear?

All methods of treatment are basically directed toward helping air to pass easily to and from the middle ear. This occurs naturally when the Eustachian tube opens or can be accomplished artificially by making an opening in the eardrum. If the cause of an improperly functioning Eustachian tube can be determined and corrected so that it opens normally, severe or permanent hearing problems in many children can be prevented because fluid will no longer form.

Simple cases are often managed medically by the judicious use of nose drops, decongestants or antihistamines, and various methods of intermittently forcing air into the middle ear (ear popping). For example, if infection within the nose or sinuses is causing nasal tissue swelling which blocks the opening of the Eustachian tube, antibiotics may prove beneficial in helping the inside of the nose to become more normal.

In other patients a surgical approach is necessary which entails the removal of infected adenoids (and tonsils in some patients) or any tissue blocking the Eustachian tube opening. Others are helped if air is temporarily able to pass freely into the middle ear by way of tiny open plastic tubes which are inserted through the eardrums.

If a child responds poorly to the above methods of management, it could indicate his basic problem is allergy causing either swelling within the nose or possibly within some portion of the middle ear. This type of patient is best helped by allergy treatment.

### Do tubes placed through children's eardrums help?

Yes. They allow air to enter the middle ear and ventilate and circulate behind the eardrums. In some patients this form of treatment, along with medical management, is essential. Unfortunately, tubes placed in eardrums tend to fall out after several (six to 12) months. When the tubes are in the eardrums, however, aeration of the middle ear is assured and hearing is temporarily restored. The tubes must be inserted carefully. The ear surgeon removes the fluid from the middle ear as he makes his opening through the eardrums (myringotomy) to insert the tubes. If the fluid is allowed to remain, it can sometimes become very thick and cause the little hearing bones located behind the eardrums to stick together so that sound cannot be transmitted normally to the inner ear. This can be a cause of permanent hearing loss.

The tubes which are inserted are of various types. Some are thin, short pieces of open plastic (Teflon) tubing which have an appearance similar to elbow macaroni which is straight and not curved. Tubes are sometimes repeatedly placed in some children's eardrums because the fluid tends to recur each time they fall out. This would indicate that the *cause* of fluid formation has *not* been eliminated. In other patients the tubes in the eardrums provide adequate aeration of the middle ear for a sufficient period of time so that the fluid problem is permanently eliminated. For example, some cases of chronic secretory otitis are due to chronic infection within the nose which has caused the tissues to swell, blocking the Eustachian tube openings. If the infection is eliminated by using antibiotics and the middle ear is well ventilated artificially via the eardrum tubes, the tissues within the nose and middle ear can gradually return to normal. In these patients, the fluid should not re-form after the plastic tubes fall out of the eardrums.

### Do tubes hurt or permanently damage the eardrums?

No. Many cases of repeated tubal insertion have been done without permanent damage to the eardrum. If, however, the tubes need to be reinserted too often, some eardrums tend to become so thin that they no longer can hold or retain a tube. Repeated unsuccessful ear "tubing" indicates that the cause of the middle ear fluid has *not* been eliminated.

### What are the disadvantages of tubes?

The major ones are:

1. Insertion of tubes requires general anesthesia and surgery.

2. Hair washing and swimming become problems. Greased knitting-wool earplugs and a tight-fitting bathing cap can be helpful if your ear specialist allows swimming. Individualized ear molds can be made. These fit well, but diving and vigorous underwater activity is often not allowed.

### Which children are most likely to have ear problems on an allergic basis?

Those who have:

1. Allergic parents or relatives.

2. Ear problems associated with nasal or other symptoms of allergies. These children often have nasal speech, and "mouth breathe."

3. Ear symptoms associated with certain pollination periods.

4. Evidence of allergies (excess eosinophilia) in their blood, nasal mucus or ear fluid.

5. Positive skin reactions to allergenic substances.

6. Persistent ear fluid in spite of repeated removal of adenoid and tonsil tissue.

### How can you tell if your child has a hearing loss?

The only accurate method is by having a hearing test performed, but the following might give you some indication that this might be needed.

1. Children often pretend not to hear their parents when they are asked to help with a household chore or go to bed. It is significant, however, if your child does not hear you when you are calling him about something he wants, such as at mealtime, or when a friend wants him to play.

2. Does your child always speak too loudly? Children often play music and the television loudly, so this would not necessarily be an indication of a hearing problem.

3. Does he indicate that he can't hear on the phone or when you speak to him in normal tones? Have friends complained that your child answers the phone and then hangs up? This often happens when the caller can't be heard.

4. Try putting your watch near your child's ear and note if he can hear the ticking when his eyes are closed.

### How are allergies which affect the middle ear treated?

If the middle ear fluid is caused by allergic tissue swelling, antihistamines may help temporarily by decreasing this swelling.

Some patients' ear symptoms can be relieved on a more permanent basis solely by making the affected child's home, in particular his bedroom, allergy-free. (See Chapter 8.)

Other children are relieved by various diets which omit the allergenic food which causes the nasal or, possibly, middle-ear tissues to swell.

Lastly, there are children who improve after they receive allergy extract-injection therapy, often in conjunction with changes in home and diet.

### If a child has a poor hearing test in school, does it mean he has ear-tube allergies?

This is possible, but the most common cause of a poor response to a routine hearing test is that the child has a cold or a nasal infection which could frequently cause a temporary hearing loss. Excess ear wax can also be a factor. Confusion sometimes occurs because the child did not understand the test.

### Can hearing loss associated with ear-tube allergies affect schoolwork?

It certainly can. Hearing loss, especially if it is minimal, can be quite difficult for a parent to detect. In school, such a loss can result in not hearing directions properly, and only the alert, interested teacher or a routine school hearing test might lead to detection of the true problem.

### If a child has a one-sided hearing loss, how can you improve his schoolwork?

Talk to his teacher and request that your child sit on the far right or left side of the room so that the "good" ear can always hear the teacher's voice.

**How can you help your physician detect a hearing problem in your child?**

When a child's hearing is being tested with tuning forks, the youngster must understand the meaning of the words "louder" and "softer." Many times you can teach this to your child, and thus aid the physician, so that the tuning fork tests are more reliable. Make a very loud sound and tell your child that this is loud. Make a softer sound and tell him this is soft. Do this several times. Then make two sounds, one after another, and see if your child can tell which is softer or louder.

**Which allergenic substances are most apt to cause ear allergies?**

Dust, molds, pets (cats), feathers, kapok and foods; the latter include milk, corn, peanuts, wheat, eggs, chicken and chocolate. Exposure to some substances such as cats, feathers or certain foods occasionally can cause sudden ear symptoms.

**Are skin tests positive if children have a hearing loss due to allergy?**

Not always. Although at times the skin test reactions to allergenic substances are similar to those seen in patients who have asthma or hay fever, in general, the skin reactions in patients with ear allergies tend to be much less strongly positive. The correlation between positive skin test reactions and ear allergy is also not as reliable as in other patients who have allergies. The reason for this discrepancy is not known. Curiously, some patients who have a hearing loss on an allergic basis may have only slightly positive skin test reactions to dust, for example, yet they seem to respond well when treated with extracts of this substance.

**Are indications for a tonsillectomy and adenoidectomy different in a child who has allergies?**

The indications for a tonsillectomy and adenoidectomy are essentially the same for any child. A child who has hay fever, however, should probably not have his tonsils removed during the pollen season (early April through October[1]) because asthma has occasionally been noted to begin in some children if this is done. If a child has hearing problems, tonsillectomy and adenoidectomy are often recommended prior to evaluation by an allergist because this treatment may restore normal hearing. Usual indications for a tonsillectomy and adenoidectomy are:

    1. Frequent, severe tonsil infections.

---

[1] See pp. 278–281 for other areas. This refers only to New York State.

2. Inability to swallow because of the size of the tonsils or noisy, difficult breathing because of large adenoids. (Children's tonsils and adenoids normally increase in size until about the age of ten, and then they tend to become smaller in size during the next few years.)

3. An abscess, *i.e.*, a localized area of pus behind or around tonsillar tissue.

4. Recurrent or permanent hearing loss.

The final decision about your child's adenoids and tonsils should depend upon the opinion of your pediatrician or family physician and the ear, nose and throat specialist.

For some strange reason, some parents are extremely anxious to have their child's tonsils and adenoids removed. Tonsils and adenoids are functional, useful tissues and, even though they are not essential, they should never be removed without adequate justification. Any surgical procedure can be complicated by some unexpected happening, and decisions in this regard should not be made lightly.

### Can dizziness, or vertigo, be caused by allergy?

This can be seen in children or adults who have an inner ear allergy which affects their sense of balance. This is at times associated with buzzing noises, a blocked ear, nausea, vomiting, emotional upsets and fatigue. Ménière's syndrome is at times localized to one side. Food allergies are occasionally found to cause this problem. Dust, pollen, chemical odors and molds can be factors.

# CHAPTER 3

# Allergic coughing and bronchial asthma

## ALLERGIC COUGHING

**What causes an allergic cough?**

Many children cough excessively for days, weeks or years prior to their initial wheezing episode. This cough is possibly caused by a slight spasm of the air tubes or by excessive lung mucus. Coughs, if caused by allergy, can sometimes be helped by giving the child an antiasthmatic medicine. This type of cough is often worse when the child exercises or is emotionally upset (as with anger or laughter), at night and when it is damp.

**What common types of cough are not caused by chest allergies?**

1. At times, children have a "throat-clearing" cough. This can be due to postnasal mucus, and an antihistamine or nose drops can be helpful in drying the mucus so that it does not cause symptoms. It is often worse at night and can cause some children to "cluck." This type of cough becomes less severe when the patient exercises. It is often caused by nasal allergies.

2. This is in direct contrast to a cough associated with asthma which is precipitated or made worse by exercise or exertion. An asthma medicine such as Bronkolixir (no prescription required) often helps this type.

3. Children with an infection, such as a cold, can frequently have a tickle in their throats causing a cough which is lessened when the infection is treated. This type of cough is at times easy to confuse with an allergic cough. Antibiotics help this. A sinus or chest X-ray and blood examination may help in diagnosing infection.

**Does the sound of an allergic cough differ from other coughs?**
Many mothers can tell the difference between the so-called "allergic" cough and an infection-type cough, the latter being much deeper, hoarser or barky in nature (like a dog's bark).

**Are all allergic coughs associated with asthma?**
No. Some children never wheeze but have a cough as their sole manifestation of allergy. A few of these children frequently have a poor response to any medicine and improve only when they have received adequate treatment with the proper allergy extract.

Many children wheeze when they cough but neither the child nor the parent realizes it.

## PROGNOSIS, DIAGNOSIS, AND TREATMENT OF ASTHMA

**What is asthma?**
Asthma is wheezing. Wheezing can be caused by many medical problems other than allergy, but the most frequent cause (after the age of two) is allergic swelling of the lining of the air tubes in the lungs and spasm or shrinkage of the muscle around the air tubes. This decreases the size of the air tubes, so that air whistles or squeaks as the child breathes out. When a child wheezes, the lungs usually also produce more mucus than normal and this adds to the chore of breathing. Asthma is usually characterized by difficulty in breathing out, although severely ill children may also have difficulty breathing air into their lungs. Infections in young children frequently cause swelling of the inside of the air tubes and this can mimic allergic asthma.

**Is all wheezing due to asthma?**
No. There are many other causes and this is the reason you should see a physician to be certain that the cause of the wheeze is allergic. In the first two years of life in particular, wheezing can be caused by many problems other than allergies. It is very important to be sure that some foreign object did not accidentally get into the child's lung tubes during a choking episode. Not all swallowed objects are revealed by an X-ray. Metallic substances, plastic or bone can be seen, but foods such as peanuts could not. Wheezing can be caused by anything which could press against the outside of the air passageways, causing an indentation within the breathing tubes, or by anything inside the air tubes obstructing the easy passage of air.

**At what age does asthma first occur?**

It can start very early in infancy. The initial episode often is noted in association with an infection such as measles, influenza, pneumonia or whooping cough. Children who wheeze often have a history of having had bronchiolitis during infancy. Atopic dermatitis or eczema during the first year of life and mild "constant colds," which are in fact allergic nasal symptoms, often precede the initial asthmatic episode. Asthma can, however, begin at any age, even in late adulthood.

**Is asthma more common in girls or boys?**

Asthma is two or three times more frequently noted in boys than in girls, prior to puberty. After this time, girls are more likely to wheeze.

**What are the common allergenic causes of asthma?**

Seasonal wheezing which occurs for one to several weeks in the spring, summer or fall is mainly due to tree, grass or weed pollens and mold spores.

Wheezing which occurs throughout the year, either sporadically or daily, is referred to as perennial. This can be due to a multitude of allergenic substances, including house dust, kapok, wool, feathers, animal hair or dander, furniture stuffing, cottonseed, flaxseed, scented substances, mold spores (in damp homes), foods and chemical odors.

Foods most apt to be factors associated with daily asthma are those eaten daily such as milk, wheat, eggs, chocolate, corn, peanut butter, citrus fruits or juices, potatoes and tomatoes. (See Chapter 9 and p. 272.) In particular, chocolate and peanut butter cause wheezing in children who eat these foods often. Foods not eaten daily which might cause occasional asthma are mustard, buckwheat, celery, certain spices, fresh berries or melon.

Many children have mild to severe intermittent or daily asthma most of the year but at certain times during the warmer months it can become much worse. These children have certain substances causing perennial symptoms, while allergenic pollens or mold spores contribute to their additional difficulty during certain seasons.

Infection, at any time of the year but particularly in the winter, may cause asthma. Emotions, fatigue, irritating odors (smoke, chemicals) and infection often seem to trigger asthmatic episodes.

**How can you tell if your child is wheezing?**

Parents can determine this as follows: Open your own mouth and breathe deeply in and out, so that you make *no noise except for the sound of the air* as it passes in and out of your mouth. The sound you hear when you do this is the same sound you should hear when you listen to anyone's normal chest. Now put your ear next to your child's naked chest or back and ask him to take similar (quiet) deep breaths through his open mouth while you pinch his nostrils closed. Be certain your child is not making throat noises when he tries to do this. If you hear a rattle or whistle as he breathes, especially as he exhales, it indicates some obstruction or blockage to breathing and this could be a wheeze. Allergic wheezing *always* affects both lungs. If you hear wheezes repeatedly only in one lung, check with your physician. Something unrelated to allergy might be blocking the exit of the air from that one lung.

Many parents believe that their child is wheezing because he squeaks or is noisy as he breathes. This is often caused by the sounds which are produced from breathing through a partially plugged nose, and is unrelated to asthma or wheezing. It is essential that you determine if the whistle is coming from the nose or from the chest. If you follow the suggestions in the previous paragraph, you should be able to make this distinction. Of prime importance is that the nose *must* be closed when you listen to your child's breathing, otherwise you may be confused by the nasal sounds heard in the lungs, or transmitted to the lungs.

### Do children outgrow asthma?

Yes. Some children certainly wheeze a few times and never again, but far too many children are allowed to wheeze for years, while everyone waits for them to "outgrow" it or to become older before having allergy tests. During this period the child cannot run, play or sometimes go outside. Parents are often amazed at the degree of improvement caused in a few days or weeks by diet, or changes in their home, or in a few short months of allergy-extract treatments. Boys often improve spontaneously at puberty while girls can sometimes become worse. Starting proper allergic management when the asthma first becomes a recurrent problem gives an infant or child the best chance of having an enjoyable, more normal childhood.

### What percentage of asthmatic children improve on treatment?

Most children who receive complete and proper allergy evaluation and injection therapy respond well. Their attacks become less severe and occur less often. Some children stop wheezing completely after several months of treatment. Usually, however, years of treatment are required. A few patients, perhaps five or ten per cent, will not respond well and will require vigorous, constant supervision and help.

### Once a child responds to treatment, does the asthma stop?

The asthma seldom stops suddenly, never to recur again. The attacks gradually become less frequent and less severe when children begin to improve. Parents are often very discouraged because their child will not wheeze for several months and suddenly a wheezing episode occurs. They are naturally fearful that the original asthmatic problem is recurring. It is the total, yearly picture which counts. The attacks should be decreasing each year. Gradual steady improvement is the allergist's aim.

### How should you treat an asthma attack?

The best solution is to prevent its occurrence by avoiding known offenders (pets, dust, foods). At times this is not possible. Allergy-injection treatments are then given and these should eventually help decrease the number and intensity of attacks. Until then, the following measures could prove helpful:

1. If the asthma is severe, put your child to bed in his allergy-free bedroom. Do not allow him to eat foods which seem to make his allergies worse. Start asthma medicine at the very first sign of asthma. Frequently this is a cough, throat-clearing or, in some children, puffy eyes or a look that only a mother can recognize. The longer the delay before starting the medicine, the longer it may take to control a wheezing episode. The medicine, if used properly, will not hurt your child. Repeated asthma which persists for years will be injurious.

Parents often delay in giving asthma medicine to treat an attack because the child is due to see the physician and the parents want the doctor to hear their child wheeze. This should never be done unless specifically requested. Consider asthma a very bad habit; prevent it whenever possible.

2. Give asthma medicine in the dose the doctor recommended and *at the time interval* recommended. Medicines are like a gallon of gasoline in a car: they last only so long. Most are effective for four to six hours, but some, which should be used mainly at bedtime, last from eight to ten hours. The shorter-acting medicines are best for effective daytime control. If the attack is severe, give the medicine every four hours. If the attack is mild, a dose of medicine every six hours should be adequate. If you are late with each dose of medicine, the air tubes can go into spasm again and this can prolong an asthmatic episode.

3. Continue medicine until the attack has subsided completely. If you have listened to the chest and heard no wheezes, whistles or squeaks for 24 hours, then it is safe to taper off or to stop the asthma medicines. Do not be so cautious that you never stop the medicines.

This is the other extreme. If school is a worry, try tapering off or stopping the medicine on weekends first. Children seldom worry about a wheeze in school. It is the parents who fear that if they don't give the medicine their child may begin to wheeze and be seriously ill by the time he arrives home. As this sometimes happens, they are justified in their fears.

### Should a wheezing child be sent to school?
(See p. 246.)

### How can you taper off the amount of asthma medicine your child is using?

First stop the middle-of-the-day dose, then the morning and lastly the night dose. If you feel your child might wheeze if the night medicine is not given, try giving one-half the usual dose for two or three nights. If your child continues to do well, stop the medicines in this gradual manner. If your child begins to wheeze again when you are attempting to decrease the amount of medicine he is using, resume the medicine in the usual dosage until you can check with your physician.

### How can you determine what is causing a *sudden,* infrequent episode of wheezing?

Some children don't wheeze very often but an alert mother will notice that she can tell from how her child acts or looks, a few hours before the episode begins, that severe asthma will occur. This type of attack is caused by something different and unusual which has occurred shortly before the warning symptoms were noted. Most often it would be an infection and this type of attack often can be aborted by immediately starting the asthma medicine and having a physician examine the child. In other patients, there does not seem to be an infection and in these cases the mother must try to recall as many of the details as possible concerning the few hours previous to the attack. Make a list of *exactly* what your child ate or placed in his mouth, where he played, what he touched or smelled, and whatever was unusual in the air during this period. Study of records after several episodes will often reveal the exact cause. Asthma attacks which occur during pollen seasons are most often caused by pollen exposure. Often, however, there are contributing factors, such as eating melon or bananas during the ragweed season, or having an infection which, combined with the pollen contact, causes a most severe wheezing episode.

**How fast should a child breathe?**

Infants normally breathe at a rate of about 30 to 40 breaths per minute; children usually breathe at a rate of about 20 to 25. If a respiratory rate is consistently over 50, contact your physician. If it is less, but you are very concerned because your child is in distress, contact your physician.

**How can you count your child's respirations?**

Using a watch or clock with a second hand, count the times your child breathes in and out in one full minute. Be careful to count the entire breath, in *and* out, as only one. If your child is wheezing badly, you can easily hear the breathing. There will generally be a slight pause after the long maneuver of breathing out. If there is only a slight wheeze, or if the child is breathing very fast, you may have to watch the abdomen go up and down. Again, one up-and-down motion is only a count of one. If your child is talking or crying, you cannot accurately count the respirations.

**Is it serious if a wheezing child's face turns white?**

Not necessarily, because this is often seen, especially if the child has just received an injection of Adrenalin (epinephrine). Children who are wheezing badly frequently have a white face, clammy, cold skin and somewhat blue lips and fingernails. Contact your physician if you observe this condition.

**Do asthmatic children perspire in excess?**

When children wheeze severely they often perspire so heavily that their hair is wet, but this subsides once the attack is under control. Many normal boys, in particular, tend to perspire to excess. Often this trait is found in the male members of a family. It is sometimes related to a food sensitivity and subsides after an allergy diet.

**How important is it if a child's lips turn blue?**

A child who is wheezing can have blue lips and nails and this usually indicates that he is not getting enough oxygen into his blood. Your physician should be contacted when this occurs.

Many children have blue lips after swimming, especially if they are chilled or overtired. This usually responds to a rest and some warmth and is unrelated to allergies.

## Can a child wheeze without knowing it?

Of course. It depends upon the degree of the asthma, and also upon the individual. Some older children are not aware when they are wheezing moderately, while some very young children can detect the slightest spasm.

## Should you ever give asthma medicines if your child is not wheezing?

Yes. If exercise or exertion, emotional upsets (happy or sad) or infections frequently cause asthma, then start asthma medicine in advance or at the very first sign of difficulty. Children should be allowed to play normally, but asthma medicine should be given before play *if asthma always or usually follows exertion.* If your child wheezes on holidays or birthdays, give medicines the day before and the day of the holiday. If you are to visit a relative who has a pet which causes your child's allergies, a new asthma medicine, Intal, might prevent an attack. (See pp. 211–212.)

If reprimands cause asthma, medicate your child first and 20 minutes later discipline your child as any other child in that age group. If you don't, you will have a spoiled child and perhaps behavior problems in the other children. Once the child has responded well to allergy treatments, this precaution is usually not necessary.

Some girls wheeze during each menses (and women during each pregnancy), which could be caused by an endocrine imbalance. Give asthma medicines (if these help) before and during menses, if this always happens.

## Why is it so very important for the asthmatic child to drink fluids when wheezing?

Mainly because much liquid is lost from the body during an asthma attack. The mucus which normally forms in the lungs must be kept thin so that it can be coughed up and spit out or swallowed. If it remains in the lungs and becomes thick and rubbery, the problem of breathing is greatly increased. Most children will not eat when asthma is severe, but they absolutely must drink. If it is not possible for them to do so, fluids may have to be given intravenously in the hospital.

Remember that a moist tongue is one of the best common signs that your child has enough fluids within his body. If the tongue seems slightly dry or sticky, more liquids must be given; if they are not accepted or cannot be retained, contact your physician.

**Which fluids are best to give to a wheezing youngster?**

Give any liquid that will be taken but will not make him worse (as cold liquids sometimes do). Give the fluids at least once an hour and give at least ½ to one cup each time, whenever the child is awake. If the child is sleeping and awakens at night, give a large glass of water in addition to the necessary medication. (Never unnecessarily awaken any asthmatic child who is sleeping quietly because if he is disturbed coughing and wheezing occur.) If cold liquids make the asthma worse or cause coughing, use soup, tea, a warm soft drink or diluted, liquid Jell-O. If cold liquids do not seem to make your child's asthma worse, give ice cream, Jell-O or half a popsicle every half hour. It is doubtful that milk causes thick mucus, except possibly in the milk-allergic child. If your child's asthma is due to chocolate, do not give your child cola drinks, because chocolate and cola are similar. Also avoid dyed beverages, apple, grape, sugar or citrus, if any of these are a problem.

**Do cold foods or liquids cause asthma or allergic coughing?**

Yes. In *some* children, a gulp of outside cold air or a gulp of an iced liquid or ice cream can cause immediate symptoms and these contacts should be avoided until treatment can be given by an allergist. After adequate therapy most children can tolerate cold foods or drinks and eventually most can tolerate cold outside air. The latter takes a longer period of treatment. To avoid the problem of cold air, urge your child to breathe with his mouth closed when outside, so that the air is warmed by passing through the nose prior to reaching sensitive lung tissues. Cover the nose with an odor-free cotton scarf.

**Does asthma cause vomiting?**

This is frequently noted, especially in younger children. Asthma causes increased mucous production in the lungs. This mucus is carried by tiny hairs, called cilia, which line the lung tubes. The mucus is normally moved toward the mouth and then swallowed. This mucous movement occurs constantly in normal persons and this aids in keeping the lungs clear of foreign particles. In asthmatics there is an excess of mucus. Children under about seven years of age usually do not spit, so they tend to cough the mucus up and swallow it. If they do this, it frequently accumulates in the stomach and causes nausea or vomiting. When a child vomits, this may cause temporary relief from the asthma, because mucus from the lungs and from the stomach is expelled. Always observe the color of the mucus. If it is cloudy white or colorless, this is normal. If it is green or yellow, this could indicate infection and probably an antibiotic will be required. Have your child thoroughly examined by your physician to be sure. Asthmatic children sometimes vomit in cars. Carry an appropriate container.

### Can vomiting be serious in asthmatics?

Yes. If it is excessive, it can lead to a dangerous fluid loss. Contact your physician if there is any concern. Certain asthma medicines such as theophylline (see p. 210), if given in an overdose, can cause vomiting of a coffee grounds-colored material and this can be a serious problem, especially if theophylline continues to be given to such a child.

### What helps to decrease the abdominal discomfort associated with asthma?

A cola beverage will often help to "settle the stomach." Add sugar or water to the cola to eliminate the bubbles or gas. Do not give cola if there is an allergy to chocolate. A hot-water bottle on the abdomen may help. Sometimes the discomfort is great. If you purposely cause your child to gag by putting a finger down his throat, this may cause him to vomit and thus help relieve the asthma and bellyache. If you do this, be careful that the child does not choke and that the vomited material does not enter his lungs. If the abdominal pain is persistent or severe, contact your physician.

### Which complications of asthma require a physician's attention?

1. Pneumonia is the most frequent problem and requires treatment with the appropriate antibiotic as soon as possible. A fever over 101° F. (38.4° C.), the presence of green or yellow mucus, an extreme amount of coughing or an increasing difficulty in breathing can indicate an infection such as pneumonia or bronchitis. Asthma medicines, although given properly, usually will *not* help to relieve this type of wheezing until the infection has also been treated. Patients who have pneumonia often cough so excessively that the wheeze is overshadowed by this symptom. It is possible to have pneumonia and not to have any fever. If the opening to a small area of the lung is plugged with mucus, the lung area collapses because no air can enter. This is called atelectasis and can be confused with pneumonia on an X-ray.

2. The lung is similar to a large, sponge-like balloon. Occasionally, when a child has coughed or wheezed very hard, a bubble forms on the outside of the balloon-like lung, and when this breaks the lung can partially collapse. When this occurs it can cause *sudden, very severe chest pain* and marked breathing difficulty associated with blue lips and nails. This is called a pneumothorax. Contact your physician or go to

the nearest hospital. A child's chest may ache or be sore from wheezing severely, but extreme pain is unusual.

3. Occasionally, air escapes from the lungs through a tiny bubble similar to a slow leak in a tire. The lung does not usually collapse to any great degree. As the air escapes, however, it accumulates under the skin so that it can be felt. The skin in the area of the upper chest near the collarbone and lower neck feels like crinkled paper. The sensation can be simulated by placing a towel over wrinkled, crushed tissue paper which has been smoothed out. As you press the paper through the towel with your fingertips, it feels similar to the tiny bubbles of air under the skin.

### What attitude should parents assume toward their child's asthma?

They should assume that the medicines or physician will help their child. Undue anxiety is contagious and can contribute to a child's breathing problems. Parents should not look frightened or act flustered.

A parent does not have to express any concern in words for a child to realize that he is upset. By merely looking calm and confident, you can relax your child and ease his breathing. Many children breathe better as soon as a physician enters the room and before any medication has been given. They realize that they are about to be helped and this alone relaxes them. A parent can convey a similar confidence and assurance.

### How can you tell when your child's asthma seems to be improving?

If a child is talking, smiling, able to lie flat and is hungry, the asthma attack is probably subsiding.

### How can you tell when asthma is so severe that you need a physician immediately?

This is difficult to answer, but if you have given asthma medicines and in 15 or 30 minutes your child is still gasping for breath, the child should be seen by a physician. If the asthma is severe, the skin seems to be "sucked-in" between the ribs and around the collar bone. A child with truly severe asthma will not eat, talk, smile or joke. His face has an anxious expression. His major and sole concern is breathing and he sits hunched forward, often with his hands on his knees, and his neck appears to be pulled in because his shoulders are raised. When he breathes it is noisy and breathing out, in particular, is difficult. His face is generally pale and moist. If the lips seem blue or the child complains of a distressing chest pain, a physician should be notified. A chest can ache from the muscular exertion of prolonged wheezing, but any sudden, *severe* pain always must be investigated.

### Can a child die from asthma?

This would be a most rare occurrence, but it can happen, despite highly efficient and successful present-day methods of treatment. If your child has severe allergies, it is imperative that you obtain the help of a well trained allergist.

### What do you do when you can't contact your physician and your child is wheezing badly?

Contact another physician or take your child to the emergency room at the nearest large hospital.

## SPECIAL PROBLEMS RELATED TO ASTHMA

### What is a normal temperature for a child?

Rectally, the temperature should be 99.6° F. (37.5° C.), *but* there is a normal range during the day from 98.6° to 100.6° F. (37°–38.1° C.). Orally, the temperature should be 98.6° F. (37° C.). Again, there is a normal variation of 1° F. so that 97.6° to 99.6° F. (36.5°–37.5° C.) may be considered normal. Low temperatures are seldom of concern. A rise of 1° F. is often not serious. If the temperature rise is 2°–3° F. (ca. 1° C.) above normal, the problem is probably not allergy, but infection. Contact your child's physician. Remember that some children can be very ill and not have a fever, even though they may have an infection such as pneumonia. Uncomplicated allergies usually do not cause high fevers.

### What is an infection?

An infection is an illness caused by various types of germs such as bacteria or viruses. The most common is a cold or upper respiratory tract infection. Other common ones affect the tonsils, throat, ear, chest or intestines. If a child is not well or if his asthma is not responding to the medicines which frequently control it, your physician should examine him to see if an infection is present.

It is certainly possible to have an infection and not be able to determine where it is. A throat infection, for example, can cause fever when the throat appears normal. Hours after the fever begins the throat may become quite red, but an examination of the throat before the redness appeared would make diagnosis very difficult. Most children have about four infections a year.

### Does an X-ray always reveal a lung infection?

Usually an X-ray would reveal an infection, such as pneumonia, but this is not always true. There are times, especially early in an infection, when the physician can hear the pneumonia but the X-ray does not show evidence of it. It is possible that a few days later the X-ray will reveal the pneumonia, but the physician might not be able to hear it at that particular time.

### Do infections cause asthma or does asthma cause infections?

Both can be true under certain circumstances. There is little doubt that allergy and infection frequently occur at the same time in some children. Allergies can cause the mucous membranes to swell, thus making a child more prone to infection and this in turn triggers the asthma. Once allergies are well treated, excessive infections are usually not noted and are much less likely to trigger asthmatic episodes. This is because the tissues are more resistant to germs or bacteria that are normally present in a child's mouth and nose. Infection can precipitate asthma but does not really cause it. It is similar to having a gun loaded with bullets. The bullets cause the allergy. Pulling the trigger, as infection does, causes no difficulty unless the bullets are there. In persons without allergies, there are no bullets. If you note that some infections of the tonsils, throat or ear, as well as common colds and flu, etc., cause asthma, then you should start asthma medicine at the very first sign of infection. Start it even before a wheeze or cough is noted, to try to prevent an asthma attack. Once children begin to wheeze with infections, most subsequent infections will cause asthma and every effort should be made to prevent this from occurring. If each such asthmatic episode is treated with an asthma medicine and if the infection is treated with an antibiotic or infection medicine, the attacks will generally be shorter and less severe. The sooner *both* medicines are started, the better. Once the allergies are well controlled by comprehensive allergy therapy, this special precaution is usually no longer necessary. Only your physician can determine if the use of antibiotics is indicated. For example, viral infections are not directly helped by antibiotics. The degree and location of a bacterial infection will alter the number of days during which an antibiotic is needed and the type of antibiotic used. Be sure to check with your doctor *before* you discontinue any antibiotic, especially if the mucus continues to be green or yellow. Such decisions can only be determined by the physician's thorough physical examination. Children who have asthma require more frequent and earlier medical examinations for slight health problems than do most children.

Some children are believed to be allergic to bacteria or a substance these organisms produce and this type of patient is often difficult to treat. An attempt may be made to treat each infection with an antibiotic (unless the doctor feels it is a viral infection), but the usual allergy extracts probably would not be recommended. Treatment with a respiratory or bacterial vaccine can be beneficial in some of these children. Although the effectiveness of these vaccines is very controversial, some allergists are impressed with the improvement noted after their use.

### Which measures can you take in your home to help diminish infections?

The following measures may not truly decrease the number of infections in your family, but they may help and are worth trying:

1. Be certain that each person in the family has his own drinking glass, or use throw-away paper cups.

2. Rinse your dishes with boiling water if someone in your family has an infection.

3. Teach children to cover their mouths when they cough or sneeze and to wash their hands frequently when they have an infection.

4. Have a child who is very prone to throat infection gargle with a mouth wash (such as Colgate 100) at least twice a day.

5. Some doctors believe that using nose drops (for example, Neo-Synephrine) (see pp. 39 and 209) and antihistamines (see pp. 207–208 and p. 275) for two or three days at the very first sign of an infection helps to abort the episode.

6. Try 250–500 mg. Vitamin C at least three to six times daily. If diarrhea indicates the dose is too high, discontinue the Vitamin C until it stops. Then resume the Vitamin C in a lower dosage.

7. A word of caution should also be added in relation to infections which develop in other members of a family when an asthmatic child is well. If your wheezing youngster always becomes ill when anyone in the family is sick, it is imperative that the sick member be isolated *completely* from the rest of the family or be treated for his infection. A mother, for example, can develop an obvious infection, such as a sore throat or severe cough which she subdues without antibiotics but, because the infection lingers for a few days, the asthmatic child suddenly develops severe asthma associated with symptoms similar to his mother's. These episodes often could have been prevented by speedy treatment of the parent at the first sign of illness.

**Should concerned parents overprotect asthmatic children?**

The answer would depend upon the definition of overprotection. If your child wheezes every time he goes outside your home, it does not take long before the child is overprotected and not allowed to play outdoors. If each time your child becomes chilled he develops an infection and then wheezes, a mother quite understandably starts to "overdress" her child. This is not overprotection but common-sense adjustment to a difficult situation. These same parents will allow normal play and normal dressing once they see that their child no longer has allergic symptoms.

If a mother continues to overdress her child or to give medicine when there is no reason for it, this is being too protective. Have your physician set up the guidelines for you to follow. He will change them when there is a reason to do so.

**Can parents make their child's asthma worse?**

Yes. Many parents are frightened by asthma. It is alarming to see your youngster gasp to breathe. But if a parent trembles, can't talk and appears to be about to cry, this will make a child worse. Any child can sense a parent's fear by the tone of voice or a slight facial change. If you have ever truly been frightened yourself, you know that you can barely breathe in and out. A wheezing child already has this difficulty, and if you add fear to this situation it is greatly worsened. You can best help your child by remaining calm and giving proper medicine. Call your physician or take your child to the hospital if you are concerned.

**Can emotions truly cause asthma?**

There is some controversy regarding this but many physicians feel that, like an infection, emotional upsets trigger asthma attacks but do not actually cause them. Tension, fatigue, exertion, chilling and smoke of any sort are also felt to be trigger mechanisms. Once a child has responded well to allergy treatment, emotions (or infection) are much less apt to be associated with asthma.

**Can asthma cause emotional problems?**

Asthma, with all its possible restrictions and limitations, can cause emotional problems for some children. In these patients, it is the asthma that causes the emotional problem and not the reverse. Thus, many psychological problems resolve themselves once the child's asthma begins to respond to an allergist's treatment. Some children with severely limiting wheezing, such as that seen in any child with a chronic illness (for example, diabetes), may need special help from a psychiatrist in accepting their disease.

### What can you do if your child is wheezing and seems to be so upset that he is making his asthma worse?

Sedatives or medicines which cause drowsiness are to be avoided as much as possible. It sometimes helps to lessen anxiety if the child is given two to three teaspoonsful of wine or whiskey in grape juice or orange juice, sweetened to taste. Needless to say, this should not be used to excess and it would be best if the child were told only that this was "medicine" to help relax him.

### How can a mother handle the child who purposely triggers an asthma attack?

There are many children, even young ones, who will state that if they are not given whatever they demand they will wheeze, and then proceed to carry out their threat. The solution to this problem is to give asthma medicine promptly, wait about 20 minutes for it to help, and then treat the child as you would any other youngster without asthma. In situations requiring immediate discipline, the waiting period can be eliminated.

Denial of what the child likes, in the form of play or food, will often be much more effective than physical punishment. Do not make idle threats which you cannot enforce, or your child will continually be challenging your authority. The child must be taught that his disease cannot be used as a threat. Unless any tendency of this type is curbed immediately, many family problems will arise in addition to a most undesirable and serious habit pattern. A child may threaten to wheeze if his mother goes out. Once again the parent must be firm. It is wise to check with the sitter frequently; also be sure that you can be reached immediately. Once a child is well treated for his allergies, and has responded, emotions are much less likely to trigger an allergic episode.

### Do breathing exercises help asthma?

Yes, they help and are essential if a child has severe asthma of long duration. A booklet called *Breathing Control for Asthma and Emphysema* (see Appendix, p. 285) is written for adults and children. It often helps if a physiotherapist initially shows the child and his parents exactly how to do the various breathing maneuvers. You can contact a physiotherapist by calling any large hospital or children's hospital. Arrangements can usually be made to learn these exercises on an outpatient basis. Essentially, the major concern is to teach the youngster to breathe using the lower rib cage and to try to breathe out more air than is breathed in. Blowing up balloons or playing games, such as blowing a Ping-Pong ball across a table at some target, also helps because it can eliminate some of the excess air trapped in the lungs.

## Should asthmatic children play wind instruments?

Musical instruments provide a means of doing breathing exercises in a pleasantly acceptable manner. Playing any small wind instrument, under a music teacher's supervision, will help a child breathe in a more controlled and proper manner and this control can be beneficial during asthma attacks. Some years ago this type of activity was felt to be harmful, but this is no longer true.

## Is surgery a problem in asthmatic children?

The indications for the removal of a child's appendix, tonsils, adenoids or teeth are the same in allergic or nonallergic children. The following should be considered:

1. It is important that the tonsils and adenoids (see pp. 48–49) not be removed during a pollen season from a child who has nasal allergies but has never had asthma. Wheezing sometimes has been noted to occur after such an operation in some children when this type of surgery is performed between April and October. (See the pollen season in your area, pp. 278–281.)

2. A second factor is the use of steroids or cortisone. (See pp. 212–215.) If your child has received such drugs within a year of surgery, your child's physician, surgeon and anesthesiologist should be informed. It is sometimes necessary to restart cortisone so that your child has added protection because of the stress of surgery.

3. A third problem which sometimes arises is related to maintaining strict diets while in a hospital situation. This is often impossible unless a parent is present to personally supervise all foods eaten. The mistakes which occur are accidental but, because of the large number of individuals caring for patients during a 24-hour period, dietary errors seem to be particularly difficult to avoid.

4. A fourth consideration is that, occasionally, children who have not wheezed for many months will suddenly have a recurrence of asthma the very morning of surgery. To prevent this, a long-acting asthma medicine should be given prophylactically the night before surgery. This will help to ensure that your child will not wheeze the morning of surgery. If your child does happen to wheeze before or after surgery, the asthma can be controlled with long-acting injections of

epinephrine or asthma medicine given rectally if drugs cannot be taken by mouth.

Lastly, it should be mentioned that children who have allergies can at times be allergic to drugs. Any previous drug problem should be explained to the physician in charge. The anesthesiologist should specifically be told that your child wheezes so that certain drugs which might interfere with breathing, such as morphine, can be avoided.

Provided that care is taken to inform the medical and surgical staff of your child's allergic problems, you should be assured that an asthmatic child who is not wheezing will usually tolerate surgery as well as other children. Be sure the hospital room is "allergy-free." (See pp. 114–115.)

### Should asthmatic boys and girls engage in sports?

Yes. They should indulge in as much activity as they can when they are not wheezing or are having only slight asthma. The only difference between them and the average child should be that they might have to take asthma medicine before a sports activity. If a youngster wheezes badly in spite of this, exercise must be curtailed until the allergies are better controlled. If limitation of activity is necessary, young boys should learn judo, weight lifting or some body-improving activity so that they are (and feel) superior in some physical way.

Asthmatic youngsters of normal size should not diet or use diuretics to meet weight requirements for wrestling or football.

### Which occupations should asthmatic children plan to avoid?

There are many occupations which could aggravate asthma, and children who could possibly wheeze in adulthood should avoid entering these careers so that their future livelihood will not be endangered. Asthmatic youngsters should not plan on becoming veterinarians, beauticians, barbers, firemen, painters, bakers, garage mechanics, taxidermists or farmers. They must avoid occupations which would expose them to inclement weather, excess moisture, heavy air pollution, excess dust, irritating odors or occupations that are physically demanding.

### How can you help to make a severely asthmatic youngster feel superior?

If at all possible, allow your child to pursue some study which can make him feel superior either mentally, artistically or physically. If your child has artistic or musical talent, encourage it. If your child loves a mental challenge, encourage chess or bridge. If your child enjoys sports, but cannot engage in such activities as football or baseball, encourage table tennis, photography, sharpshooting, judo, karate and weight lifting. Girls may knit, crochet, sew or design clothes. Ventriloquy, magic or card tricks are other possibilities. Special lessons are helpful.

### Should asthmatic girls go to slumber parties?

If the asthma is a mild problem, such a party might not be a point of concern provided the youngster carries her own pillow and has her asthma medicine to use if necessary. If the girl's asthma is moderate to severe, there are many unforeseen problems which can arise. Such parties are often held in damp basements or dusty attics. The pillows or sleeping bags are often made of kapok or feathers. The girls stay up late and become fatigued. The combination of excitement and exhaustion, plus new allergenic exposure (frequently including pets), can precipitate an asthmatic episode./Many youngsters are reluctant, for many reasons, to tell the parents in charge of the slumber party when the wheezing begins, and the asthmatic girl will seldom call her parents during the night. By morning she may be very ill.

The best solution seems to be to allow the youngster this pleasure, provided sensible precautions are taken. These would include (1) having your child prophylactically take her asthma medicine, especially Intal, to prevent wheezing; (2) having her carry a nonallergenic pillow and sleeping bag; (3) a discussion about your child's problems with the parent in charge of the gathering; and (4) an attempt to eliminate major allergenic factors, such as pets and feathers.

### Does asthma cause emphysema?

It can lead to this problem in adults if asthma is severe and cannot be controlled. Emphysema, in simple terms, means that the small sections of the lungs, which look like a sponge, have lost their elasticity and have been broken down by infection and breathing problems. The small lung sections are enlarged and not intact, so the tissue is no longer as capable as it once was. Air cannot be forced out of the lungs effectively if the small lung sections have become enlarged; therefore, the air is trapped in these areas. Prolonged infection in asthmatics is only one cause of emphysema in adults. Children who have chronic severe asthma frequently have marked air-trapping or possibly what has been called a reversible preemphysema. True emphysema probably seldom occurs, except possibly in older adults who have wheezed severely for many years. This type of patient is often breathless when no wheeze is evident.

## Does asthma cause poor growth?

No. If, however, a child is constantly ill with infections and asthma, the growth may not be as great as when allergies are under control. Children who take daily doses of a steroid or cortisone (see p. 213) for prolonged periods of time can definitely grow more slowly than normal, but if the high doses of cortisone are stopped before the time a child normally stops growing in the late teens, a growth spurt will usually occur and normal height can be attained. If cortisone is given on alternate days rather than daily, growth will be more normal. Very low doses of certain types of cortisone do not affect growth adversely. Cortisone frequently causes a weight gain, which can be temporary or permanent. This is often most evident in the rounded face or hump on the back of the neck. In some food-allergic children, growth suddenly improves when offending foods are recognized and eliminated.

## Does asthma hurt a child's lungs or heart?

Children can wheeze many times without measurable objective evidence to show an alteration in the lungs or heart. As with any strain, asthma can make the heart beat faster, but this does not hurt the normal heart. The heart beats faster, for example, whenever any child plays actively. X-rays show no abnormality that is particularly specific for asthmatics. Only the most exceptional asthmatic child would show significant changes on an electrocardiogram.

## Does asthma cause chest deformities?

Not in most children. When a child is wheezing, excess air is temporarily trapped in the lungs and the chest may appear to be rounder than normal, but this generally subsides as soon as the attack stops. Asthma seldom causes a caved-in "funnel chest" or a prominent, convex "pigeon-chest" except possibly in an extremely ill youngster who has wheezed severely for ten or 15 years. Adults, however, who have wheezed for long periods of time can have permanently rounded or so-called "barrel" chests associated with emphysema.

## Will a move to another part of the country stop your child's asthma?

It may not. Your child's response to a move will depend upon exactly what is causing the asthma. If it is a certain food which he will eat wherever he goes, a move will not help. If the cause is something in your home, such as a comforter or a pillow, and you take it with you when you move to the new area, this will be of no help. Many patients in the East believe that a move to Denver or Arizona will solve their problems. If your child is allergic to eastern ragweed pollen, and is ill only when this is in the air in the East, a move to the West may help, but only if your child does not become allergic to the western variety of ragweed pollen. This could occur after about two years of exposure, but if a patient were fortunate it might never occur. There is some evidence to suggest that significant *new* allergies occur less often than expected when allergic patients move, but no one can predict for certain exactly how any individual patient will respond. A patient can't really move away from pollen because any area that has trees, grass or weeds will have pollen. If a patient lives in the Midwest and the pollen counts are extremely high in the area where he lives, treatment with an extract of this pollen may not be sufficiently helpful. A move to a more pollen-free area, which has much less of this aggravating substance, may definitely be beneficial for this particular patient.

A new home, new job and location, however, may only mean new problems. Most moves entail a loss of a father's place of employment, a loss of money in the move, a loss of friends and a separation from family and relatives. Before any major move for the child's sake is considered, at least two well trained allergists should agree that this is the only possible help for your child.

### Should your asthmatic child be sent to a special home for allergic children?

This is such an important decision that it would be best if two well trained allergists agreed on this before any definitive action is taken. Fortunately, it is infrequent that a child is so ill that this is warranted. Although some "difficult-to-treat" children improve under such circumstances, their problems unfortunately can persist in the special home or recur when they finally return to their own home.

These special homes for unusually severely affected asthmatic children often charge parents according to their ability to pay. There are about 20 in the United States and your allergist or the Asthma and Allergy Foundation of America can furnish more information.

### Should you have more children if you have a severely asthmatic child?

If you fear that you might have another severely asthmatic child, you should put your mind at ease. It is not uncommon to find two or even more children in one family who have allergies, but severely ill youngsters are the exception and it would be extremely unusual to have two in the same family. If two children in one family have allergies, the problems would generally not be of equal intensity or severity. Having one severely allergic child could tend to prevent or delay the onset of allergies in the siblings because your home would be allergy-free, and if problems did arise they would be realized sooner and aborted or treated more effectively.

**Can a young man be ineligible for the armed forces if asthma has been a problem during childhood?**

Yes. Wheezing beyond the age of 12 years, *if it is documented by a physician,* could make a young man unacceptable (as can a moderate or severe generalized reaction to a stinging insect or a documented allergy to wool, chronic urticaria or uncontrollable hay fever). It is indeed possible for the rigors of military life to precipitate a recurrence of asthma in a young man who has not wheezed for years.

# CHAPTER 4

# *Eczema*

**What is eczema?**

This is often called allergic or atopic dermatitis. It is a noncontagious rash which is usually very itchy. In most patients eczema is worse during the winter months. It is generally located at first on the cheeks and is noted by the age of 3 to 6 months. Later, it is located in the creases and on the outer lower parts of the legs and arms. However, it can cover the entire body. The buttocks and upper inner-arms occasionally may be spared. At times, the body lesions are coin-shaped. Frequently, the skin tends to clear without any special treatment by the age of two to three years, but these children often have dry skin the rest of their lives. Eczema persists well into adult life in about 25 per cent of severely allergic children. In older children the skin in the creases of the arms and legs and back of the neck tends to become thick and darker than normal. At puberty, eczema can change with the situation, becoming better for some patients and worse for others.

In most infants, if the skin is very soft and not dry, there is a better chance that eczema will not be a severe, prolonged problem. The term "eczema" is very general and there are many other skin rashes which denote types of eczema. These may have nothing to do with allergies. In this chapter the term "eczema" refers only to the type which is a skin allergy.

**What causes eczema, or atopic dermatitis?**

The same substances which cause other allergies are believed to be definite factors related to eczema. Such things as dust, foods, wool, some scented substances, mold spores, yeast, pollens, pet dander and hair, and feathers are examples. Foods are of particular significance in infant and adult eczema; pollens cannot be a factor until after the age of two years.

**How can eczema be prevented?**

Unless we understand what causes atopic dermatitis, or eczema, we cannot easily prevent it. Total breast feeding should be encouraged. Avoidance of factors which could obviously, or possibly, make it worse are the most effective measures. Treatment for molds, yeast, dust and foods is sometimes helpful.

### How can you obtain a clue as to what causes your child's eczema?

Watch your child while he's eating or playing. If he suddenly begins to scratch, especially in the arm or leg creases, it may indicate a recent exposure to something to which he is very sensitive. A definite rash might be evident by the next day. Subsequent purposeful exposure at some future time could confirm or deny your suspicion.

Sometimes parents note that their child's skin seems almost perfect and then, suddenly, one morning the eczema is again evident. Each subsequent day the appearance of the skin becomes worse. The answer to what may be causing the problem lies in determining what was unusual *the day before* the rash *first* appeared. Did your infant or youngster eat any new foods or engage in any different activities on that day? Was there an exposure to anything out of the ordinary? You must make a list of everything you can recall which touched your child's skin or which your child ate on *this* day. You can check your suspicions when the skin is fine again by purposely exposing your child in order to see the effect.

Although the exact mechanism by which eczema occurs is not known, it appears that eczema which appears prior to the age of one year seems to be caused in some patients by certain foods or exposure to such items as dust or wool. The allergist will try to relate any flare-up of skin problems to exposure of possible known allergenic substances, but a mother who has complete care of her infant is extremely valuable in assessing this type of history if she trains herself to be watchful. Even air pollution may cause some types of eczema.

### At what age does eczema start?

It can begin at any age and, at times, it can appear quite suddenly. Usually, however, it is first noted in early infancy.

### Do children who have eczema develop other allergies?

Yes. There is about a 50 per cent chance that a child with eczema will subsequently develop other allergies by the age of ten. Usually this will be hay fever or asthma or both. These problems possibly may be prevented by carrying out the precautions outlined in Chapter 8, or by consulting an allergist.

**How should skin medicines be applied to patients?**

You can apply a salve or cream locally as often as prescribed by your physician, dermatologist or allergist. Proper use is to apply very tiny amounts at least four times a day. Put a small amount of the salve on the end of your finger. Dab *very tiny* specks over the area of skin affected by the eczema. The specks should be about one-half inch apart. Rub the specks together. This method of application will cover the skin with an even, thin coating of salve and will more effectively and inexpensively help the skin. Using the salve as if it were cold cream is uneconomical. Most salves contain some steroid (hydrocortisone) to help diminish the rash. The problem with putting salve on the skin is that the rash returns as soon as you stop using it.

**Is cortisone safe to use in the treatment of eczema?**

When it is part of a salve and is applied to the skin, adverse effects are rarely noted.

If cortisone is taken by mouth, the eczema will usually clear up, but when attempts are made to decrease the dose or to discontinue the drug, the eczema may become worse again. For this reason cortisone is used in this form only if absolutely necessary.

**Can skin medications make the rash worse?**

Yes. If your child's skin seems to itch or burn immediately after applying salve, stop using it until your physician is notified. This problem sometimes can be eliminated by wetting the skin slightly with water prior to applying the salve. If the skin appears to be worse the day following application of a new lotion (liquid medicine) or salve, stop its usage until you have talked to your physician. It is a very wise precautionary measure to apply any new salve to an area of skin about two inches in diameter and wait 12 hours before applying it to larger areas of the body, since patients may be sensitive to some ingredient of the salve.

**How do antihistamines help eczema?**

These help by decreasing the itch or by making the patient too sleepy to scratch. If scratching is noted during the night, then a *long-acting,* eight- to 12-hour antihistamine should always be given to the child at bedtime. Many antihistamines cause children to become very sleepy and are therefore excellent to use at bedtime.

**Are allergy skin tests helpful to treat eczema?**

Yes. Traditional dust, mold and pollen tests help. Food tests are less helpful unless the newer methods are used. The upper inner-arm is usually not affected by the rash and can be used for skin testing most patients who have eczema.

### Do allergy-injection treatments help eczema?

Yes, in certain patients.

Allergy-extract treatments seem to help the type of eczema which flares up or is worse during spring and summer months when pollens and mold spores are prevalent. It does not, however, always help the more typical patient with winter eczema, although sometimes the response in such a patient is dramatic and encouraging, especially using the newer methods.

Allergy-injection treatments occasionally cause a flare-up of the eczema. This may be noted a day or two after an injection treatment. Treatment can generally be continued without causing the eczema to become worse, if the extract-injection medicine is made much weaker or the dose decreased.

### How can the itch be diminished?

1. Medicines called antihistamines (see pp. 207–208 and 275) tend to diminish an itch. On occasion, several antihistamines may have to be tried before a satisfactory one is found. These are taken by mouth. Antihistamines should not be applied directly to the skin because it is possible to cause a sensitivity to the antihistamine in the salve or lotion.

2. By applying salve which contains an anti-itch ingredient in the form of a tar. This is an ingredient which makes the salve slightly tan or dark in color.

### Does water make eczema worse?

No. Many children can swim every day all summer and their skin is not adversely affected. In general, it seems that soap or possibly the scouring powder left in a tub after cleaning irritates the skin. Showers are better than tub baths for this reason. The water temperature can cause itching if it is too hot. Tepid baths are best.

### Can some infections make a patient's eczema worse?

Yes. Colds and other viral infections may sometimes make eczema worse. Measles, paradoxically, often seems to make eczema better.

### Which body or face soap is best for a child who has eczema?

A mild soap that is neither too acid nor too alkaline. Most soaps are very alkaline. Try the more expensive hypoallergenic soaps carried in pharmacies. These include Aveeno, Basis, Lowila, Stiefel or Soydome, or a mild, regular soap such as white Dove. Certain scented soaps have an odor which bothers some patients who have allergies. Any soap that contains lanolin (or cold cream) could possibly make eczema worse because lanolin is derived from the wool of sheep. Judge a soap by trying it and watching your child's response.

### Do children with eczema improve if they "never" bathe?

Some certainly do. Certain lotions, such as Cetaphil (for which no prescription is needed), can be used to clean the skin, and some dermatologists believe that the dry skin, so typical of children with eczema, will become softer if only soap substitutes are used to cleanse the skin.

### Which laundry soap is best for a child with eczema?

A product called Safesuds, which may be purchased by the pound at your drug store, is generally most satisfactory. This soap will clean clothing but it will *not* brighten or bleach it. However, Safesuds will not leave a residue in clothing to irritate a child's skin. Safesuds seems best not only for all the child's clothing but also for towels, sheets, pillow cases or any other items which come in direct contact with the skin. If you use Safesuds for your child's white clothing, bleach them about once a month but be certain to rinse the clothing at least twice after doing this. Do not use bleach more often than absolutely necessary. Have your child wear colored clothing to decrease the necessity for bleaching. Another tip is to check the rinse cycle of your washing machine. Be certain the last rinse water looks clear. If it does not, use less soap or rerinse clothing until the last rinse water is clear. You may prefer to put the laundry through an entire extra wash-and-rinse cycle, using no soap.

### What recommendations, in relation to bathing, relieve eczema?

The major recommendation is to use as little soap as possible. Wash the areas of skin which need to be cleansed each day, but do not soap all over every day because this tends to dry the skin and causes more scratching, which makes eczema worse. In colder months, once-a-week bathing, or less, should be adequate. Bathing in water without soap may be done as often as desired. Showers are preferred to long soaks in a tub of soapy water.

Never allow your child to use bubble bath because this often contains detergents which tend to dry the skin. Young children, in an effort to produce more bubbles, often use an excess of the bubble-bath powder.

Very hot baths should be avoided because they cause overheating and this increases the tendency to itch and scratch.

**Do bath oils help dry skin?**
Putting an oil into tub water causes oil to line the tub, which makes it slippery and dangerous. If any oil is on the skin, it tends to be wiped off onto the towel. Little, therefore, actually stays on the skin and there is some doubt whether any oil that is applied really penetrates the skin.

**What special problems may arise in children or infants who have eczema?**
Infection is frequently a problem in patients who have eczema. Scratching with dirty fingernails is probably a major factor. This causes the lymph nodes or glands in the armpits or groin to become swollen and tender. At times a local antibiotic in the salve applied to a rash will help, but if infection is extensive, antibiotics may have to be taken by mouth. Be certain your child is examined by a physician if this is noted. Infection may, at times, not be the cause of a fever.

**Do children who have had severe eczema for many years have any unusual problems?**
Yes. In rare instances visual problems can be noted in some children who have had chronic severe eczema for very long periods of time (ten years or so). These are caused by cataracts. An eye physician (*i.e.,* an ophthalmologist) or an optician or optometrist can appraise this situation by a slit-lamp eye examination. Cataracts can be removed surgically by an ophthalmologist.

**Why should no child who has eczema be vaccinated for smallpox?**
No child who has eczema, or any member of this child's family, including parents, should be vaccinated until the skin of the patient is entirely clear. (The skin should be free of *any* skin rash of *any* type.)
Vaccination is no longer compulsory. If it is necessary, your physician can furnish you with a statement saying that your child cannot be vaccinated. Smallpox vaccinations are a major concern because contact with anyone who has recently been vaccinated may cause a child's eczema-affected skin to develop smallpox-like vaccination lesions. This can be a serious medical problem and is called "eczema vaccinatum." If a child who has eczema is vaccinated by error, the above usually does not occur, but if it does, a physician can obtain special vaccine and a drug to help your child. If another child in your family is acci-

dentally vaccinated, there is danger only for the child who has eczema. Be especially careful not to put a child who has eczema in a tub of water previously used to bathe a recently vaccinated youngster. The two children must be separated by having one or the other stay with a relative until the scab falls off the vaccinated area.

A new medicine which is said to be very effective and safe for vaccinating children against smallpox should be available soon for those who have eczema and who for some reason must be vaccinated.

### Can exposure to cold sores (herpes simplex) cause eczema to become worse?

Yes! The effect is similar to that of exposure to a smallpox vaccination. The areas of skin which are or have been affected by the eczema may become much worse, and the child can develop a fever and become very ill. Children who have eczema should therefore be very careful to avoid all contact with persons who have cold sores. This would include sisters, brothers or parents.

### Are there any other immunizations[1] which children with eczema cannot have?

The only precaution that should be followed is that if your child cannot eat eggs, any vaccine (such as flu vaccines) grown on egg should not be given without your physician's special recommendation. If your child can eat eggs but does not like them, or if the skin test to eggs is positive but your child has no obvious difficulty eating eggs, then the vaccine would usually be well tolerated.

Children with eczema can tolerate diphtheria, tetanus and polio protection immunization as well as any other child.

### If a patient has eczema, should he be seen by a dermatologist or an allergist?

A dermatologist is a medical specialist in skin diseases; an allergist is a medical specialist in allergies. A patient with eczema should be seen by both of these specialists because each may help with certain aspects of his problems.

The dermatologist might be better able to prescribe various preparations to be used directly on the skin. The allergist would probably be more able to help the patient determine why his skin is breaking out and could help to prevent or at least delay the onset of other allergies. Both could offer advice regarding the use of antihistamines and possible diets.

[1] See Chapter 13.

If a child has eczema and other allergies, an allergist should certainly be seen. As mentioned before, the "winter type" of eczema *sometimes* clears up to a marked degree when a child is being hyposensitized for hay fever or asthma. Eczema which becomes worse mainly during the summer is probably caused by pollen or molds, and if it is, it should be helped by extract therapy.

### What is the difference between an ointment or a cream?

An ointment is somewhat gray in color, very greasy and similar to Vaseline. A cream is whitish in color and more similar to cold cream. Creams are tolerated better than ointments by most eczema patients.

The medicine which is to help the skin is placed into either an ointment or a cream so that it can be spread upon the skin. Sometimes one seems to help a patient more than the other. Your observation concerning which helps most will aid your physician in selecting the most effective preparation for your child's skin.

### Does scratching cause or aggravate eczema?

It seems to do both. If a broken arm is in a cast, and a child is exposed to something which causes his eczema to become worse, no eczema will be found under the cast. The eczema on the opposite arm, after being scratched, will be obvious.

Allergic eczema is always itchy. A change in temperature or a slight draft can trigger the itchy sensation.

### Do children with eczema have special physical characteristics?

Yes. They often have special wrinkles under the lower eyelids called a "Dennie's sign." These are most evident if the child also has asthma and hay fever. These lines can be seen at birth and last a lifetime. In addition, children with eczema often have a pale face and very wrinkled palms.

### Which eczema infants are most apt to develop other allergies?

1. Those who have severe eczema and many allergic relatives.
2. Those who developed eczema very early in life.
3. Those who cannot eat eggs.
4. Those who have strong evidence of allergy in their blood (elevated IgE and eosinophils).

**Should a child who has eczema be kept home from school if vaccinations are being given in the school to various classes?**

Yes, if your child has severe eczema and if you want him to be entirely safe. A smallpox vaccination is considered to be contagious until the crust or scab has fallen off.

If a child has very little eczema, and the vaccinations are being given in another classroom, there should be relatively little danger for the child in school. Ask your physician's opinion in this situation.

**Can a child travel abroad if he has eczema and cannot be vaccinated?**

Yes. A child who has eczema may leave and return to the United States without a smallpox vaccination, provided that there was no travel in a country where smallpox is a problem and provided that the parents have a statement on their physician's stationery indicating why a vaccination was not performed.

Sometimes a child who has eczema and has not been vaccinated travels to a country where smallpox is present. If this child visits such a country, within 14 days of the child's return to the United States immigration officials may quarantine such a child for about two weeks.

Smallpox is presently a problem in parts of Afghanistan, Brazil, Congo (Dem. Rep.), Ethiopia, India, Indonesia, Kenya, Nepal, West Pakistan, South Africa and Sudan.

**What other nonspecific measures help eczema?**

1. Avoid overheating because this causes increased perspiration which in turn causes itching. Exertion, emotion or an overheated home or bedroom can make a child's eczema worse. Hot baths can have a similar effect. Increased home humidity may help.

2. Keep the child's fingernails short and clean to avoid damage to the skin and possible infection. The nails should be filed short twice a week so that no white shows at the outer edge or tip of the nail. Be sure there are no sharp points or jagged edges. At night it is sometimes most helpful to have the child wear mittens. No attempt should be made to tie down a child's arms and legs in his bed to prevent scratching. Older children don't want to scratch but they can't avoid doing so because their skin is so itchy.

3. Have your infant or child wear colored clothing, preferably loose-weave cottons. He should not wear wool or synthetic fabrics which might tend to cause perspiration. Not only should the patient avoid wool, but parents and relatives should also be particularly careful to

avoid wearing wool when they hold or embrace a child who has eczema. Loose-fitting clothing is better than tight-fitting shirts or pants which prevent free circulation of air about the skin. Zippered sleeping suits or warm flannel pajamas are also to be avoided. Rough fabrics of any type with animal hair or coarse fibers should not be worn. Avoid direct carpet contact.

4. A trip to a warm, dry, sunny climate often gives temporary relief.

# CHAPTER 5

# Special problems in infants under the age of one year

## Which symptoms of allergy do infants sometimes have?

1. *Digestive Problems*. Colic causes infants frequently to pull their legs up to their abdomens, and to cry and scream with abdominal discomfort. They act as if they are very hungry. (This may indicate a milk, corn, wheat or sugar allergy in infants during the first three months of life, and after that age innumerable foods may be implicated.) Excess gas, mucus, diarrhea, spitting-up and canker sores are also sometimes noted. Cereals or milk are often the cause of this problem. The need for frequent formula changes often indicates a food allergy, as does colic which lasts beyond three months.

2. *Skin Allergies*. These appear in the form of a rash called eczema or atopic dermatitis which starts on the cheeks and later is localized to the creases of the arms and legs.

The rash, at times, covers the entire body or is scattered over the body in round patches (see Chapter 4). Persistent buttock rashes may indicate allergy. It seldom is evident before the age of two months, but usually is noted before the child is six months old.

3. *Nasal Allergies*. These are indicated by the presence of watery nose mucus which does not become thick or colored yellow, green or grey, or by stuffiness without much mucus. Parents often misinterpret these symptoms and believe their infant has a slight but almost constant "cold." (See p. 38 and Chapter 2.) A frequent complaint is that they have difficulty taking their formula properly because the nose, being so swollen inside, makes it impossible for them to breathe and to suck at the same time.

4. *Disposition Problems*. Irritability, inability to sleep or reluctance to smile.

5. *Chest Allergies*. The infant experiences coughing or difficulty in breathing in and out; a chest rattle or wheeze is heard. Unlike older children, infants can remain flat when in severe respiratory distress (see Chapter 3).

6. *Infection*. Recurrent infections in infants are sometimes secondary to allergy. Infections of this type often stop when the allergies are treated. Infant ear infections may be due to milk or food allergy.

Please remember that all of the above symptoms can be caused by other problems and your infant should be thoroughly examined by your physician. For example, bronchiolitis is an infant viral infection which causes wheezing. It is very difficult to distinguish asthma from this disease. It is significant that many patients who subsequently develop asthma have a history of having had bronchiolitis in infancy.

### Which foods cause allergies in infancy?

Milk, wheat or other cereals such as corn or oats, egg, sugar or foods which contain these products (see Appendix, p. 271) are the major offenders. Eggs should be avoided for at least the first 12 months. Wheat and chicken should be withheld for the first nine months, if possible. These precautions are felt by some allergists to reduce the tendency to develop eczema, asthma and allergic nose symptoms in the allergy-prone infant. Foods are considered the major cause of any allergic symptom in an infant less than one year old.

For some reason that cannot be readily explained, if a food causing an allergy is completely omitted from the diet for several weeks, or a few months, this omission alone seems to eliminate the problem. Reintroducing the food to the diet is usually not associated with a recurrence of the symptoms.

Although rice or soybean milk, for example, are considered to be nonallergenic foods, these at times can produce any of the symptoms characteristic of allergies. See page 272 for a list of the most allergenic foods. Although it may appear that a certain food causes symptoms in infancy, allergy is not always related to the problem.

### How can you determine if your infant has a food allergy?

A physician will need to help you do the following.

*If you suspect only one food:*

You can check for individual foods by omitting the suspect food for at least five to 12 days *in all forms* (see pp. 146–165). In 12 days, or earlier if the infant seems much better, re-add the food which was omitted, in excess for one to three days, and see if symptoms recur. Infants often become irritable and fretful shortly after eating an allergenic food. You can check for any food in the manner suggested but, if a food is apt to cause serious symptoms, do not re-add it in excess but have your physician advise you on how to re-add it to the diet slowly and safely. If allergic symptoms occur each day or most days, it is probably a food that is eaten almost daily which is causing the difficulty.

*If you suspect several foods:*

The above method is helpful *only* if an infant is allergic to only one food. If several foods cause the allergic symptoms, an easy and effective method to solve this problem is to try the Rotary Diet on p. 166. Babies often drool, fret, cry and act upset shortly after they eat an offending food. Feed each of the foods allowed on each of the four days of the Rotary Diet, one at a time. Note if any symptoms occur within two to three hours. If you find that certain foods repeatedly cause symptoms, check with your doctor. He can help you make a satisfactory substitute.

If this diet proves helpful, then add one new food to the diet each day. Start with a little, early the first day, and, if there is no problem, feed your child gradually increasing amounts throughout the day. If the symptoms are not worse, then the test food is not causing difficulty and it can be eaten every fourth day as part of the infant's regular diet. If a food possibly makes the infant worse in any way, or definitely does, stop giving it for a couple of months before retrying it. (See Chapter 9 for additional necessary and helpful information.)

## What are frequent errors parents make when attempting dietary studies?

1. Be sure to read carefully all labels on *everything* you intend to feed your infant. Study the list in the Appendix on page 271, which shows unusual sources for certain foods responsible for allergies. For example, there can be milk and wheat in soup, eggs in mayonnaise and milk in margarine, etc.

2. Parents frequently believe that a little bit of the food will not affect the dietary study, so a bite of bread or cookie is given to a child when no wheat is to be eaten. Some children are so allergic to certain foods that the smallest amount which you could give them could cause symptoms for days. When dietary studies are carried out, all concerned must cooperate as fully as is possible in daily living. Mistakes and accidents will happen. Re-do the food diet from the beginning when this occurs.

3. Parents and even infants can become impatient with dietary trials but every effort must be made not to discontinue the diet in less than 12 days unless definite improvement is noted. If an infection occurs just when you are about to re-add foods, wait until the infection has subsided before any additions or it will be difficult to determine if the infection or the addition of a new food caused the symptoms.

4. Re-add eggs, wheat, corn, milk and sugar first. Restore as many other single foods to the diet as possible before adding mixtures (such as vegetables and beef).

5. For normal bone growth, infants and children need calcium and phosphorus normally found in milk. Soybean milk will give these minerals in an adequate amount. If no milk or soybean milk is taken for more than two weeks, check with your physician about a calcium and phosphorus substitute.

6. When watching for symptoms, watch everything. Any unusual complaint could be related to the food recently added. Sometimes a food causes a runny or stuffy nose, asthma, coughing, bellyaches, irritability, an eczema-like skin rash, inability to sleep, excessive drooling, reluctance to smile or any combination of these symptoms.

**Can vitamins be given during dietary studies in infants?**

They not only can but *must* be given because infants grow very quickly and need them. Vitamins should not be discontinued for more than 10 days consecutively during the first nine months of life. You can test vitamins by adding them to the basic diet as a new "food" every five days. See page 138 if you suspect vitamins of causing allergic symptoms.

**What other substances cause allergy in infancy?**

House dust (for details, see Chapter 8).

Scented substances, particularly scented body powders, diaper pail deodorizers, diaper cleaning agents, diaper liners (use non-scented Freshabyes or Flushabyes), baby lotions or creams, facial or toilet tissues, soaps, bathroom or kitchen aerosols.

Molds—Room vaporizers or humidifiers can become moldy.

Pet dander or hair—Be sure padding of the playpen is not horsehair. Also be sure the baby's mattress is synthetic or has an intact, overall plastic coating. (The odor of plastics sometimes causes allergy.)

Feathers—Infants seldom use pillows, but are sometimes in their parents' bed. If this happens, the parents' entire bedroom should be made allergy-free.

Wool—This includes blankets, clothing, contact with parents' woolen clothing and carpets.

Odors—Synthetic carpets, draperies, furniture covers or cleaning solutions.

**How can these substances which cause allergies in infancy be avoided?**

Refer to the Appendix, pages 263–268, and Chapter 8, which describe where each of these can be found. Study the directions, as outlined on page 114, on how to make your infant's bedroom as allergy-free as possible.

**Is an infant too young to see an allergist?**

No. Many infant problems can be handled quite effectively by a telephone call to the allergist after the initial detailed history and physical examination are completed. Foods are the major cause of problems and these are best studied by dietary trials and not by the usual skin tests. In an exceptional infant, a dozen or so skin tests might have to be done and many of these could be avoided by taking careful precautions in the home. The major value of seeing the allergist, however, is not only to diagnose and solve the *present* problem, but also to help prevent *future* allergic problems.

**Do infants ever need to receive extract treatments?**

Yes, but most infants are allergic to foods or other substances which can be avoided. Occasionally, an infant living in a musty, damp or dusty home might have to receive treatments for molds and dust. If recurrent infections are associated with wheezing episodes, a bacterial vaccine sometimes is helpful. This treatment is, unfortunately, no longer encouraged.

**Do infants outgrow their allergies?**

They frequently seem to "lose" their symptoms of food allergies by the time they are one or two years old. However, if they are destined to have major allergic symptoms, dust, molds and wool may cause some allergic manifestations to appear by the age of two to five years; there may be the recurrence of a previous allergic symptom such as nasal allergies, or the occurrence of a new form of allergy, such as asthma, hives, hyperactivity or chronic aches.

Pollen sensitivities do not appear until a child is at least one or two years old, since pollen exposure must occur for at least one or two years before an allergy to it becomes obvious.

**How can infant allergy be prevented?**

1. Make the bedroom as allergy-free as possible, as indicated on page 114.

2. Avoid the major substances known to cause allergies in many children, as indicated in Chapter 8 and Appendix I.

3. Avoid *ever* acquiring any pets with fur or feathers.

4. Add foods very slowly in infancy. Try to breast-feed or possibly use soybean milk rather than cow's milk preparations. When adding new foods, feed them every five days. Notice if any symptoms occur suddenly (within an hour) when the food is eaten five days later. If no allergy symptoms occur or the symptoms normally evident are not worse in any manner, that food is probably all right. When adding fruits and vegetables, add them singly, not in mixtures. Delay the addition of chocolate, nuts, peanut butter or fish, and avoid excess wheat products and orange juice. (See Rotary Diet.)

5. Vitamins are usually *synthetic* and do not cause problems, but an allergy to a certain vitamin, or to a flavor or coloring in the preparation being used, is sometimes noted. Cod liver oil should be avoided as it could possibly cause a fish sensitivity.

6. Be sure that the inside and outside of stuffed animals is cotton. If in doubt, open a seam and pull out a little of the filling. Place some of the covering and stuffing in an ash tray and burn it. If it smells like a singed chicken, it means it is of animal origin and the entire stuffing should be replaced by cotton toweling. Kapok or feather filling can cause allergies, as can the odor of polyurethane, rubber or soft plastic.

7. If there are many members in the family with serious allergies, you should consider installing an electrostatic-precipitation unit (see p. 126 ff.) in the bedroom or furnace in order to eliminate dust, mold spores and pollens. If these are removed from the bedroom, it means that the infant is less apt to become allergic to them, or at least the onset of pollen allergies may be delayed. However, the odor of these machines can sometimes make allergic symptoms worse.

### Should potentially allergic babies be breast-fed?

Yes. Although foods and drugs can pass through the milk, there is little controversy that breast-fed babies have fewer allergies than bottle-fed ones. If breast milk seems to cause symptoms, elimination of highly allergenic foods from the mother's diet may solve the problem, or the mother should go on a Rotary Diet.

### Do foods eaten while a mother is pregnant affect the baby?

Yes. Although the evidence is far from conclusive, there are occasional cases where mothers ate a great excess of certain foods, such as bananas or nuts, during pregnancy and subsequently the child had symptoms of allergies the very first time this particular food was eaten. It has been suggested that the food passed through the placenta and this allowed the infant to become allergic to it.

Many allergists recommend that no eggs, as such, be eaten during pregnancy. The pregnant mother should not drink excessive amounts of milk, should not eat cheese and should avoid excess quantities of any food. A widely varied diet is best. She must be certain to check with her physician so that she eats enough foods containing calcium and phosphorus to assure normal bone growth in her developing baby.

### Should potentially allergic infants be fed soybean milk?

The evidence to prove that this is beneficial or necessary is not completely clear. Occasionally, a baby can become allergic to soybean milk but cow's milk is more apt to be responsible for infant allergies, possibly because it is more generally consumed. If every effort is being taken to avoid allergies from developing in an infant, *the baby should be breast-fed*. If this is impossible, then the infant should be fed soybean milk. Common brands sold in drug stores are Sobee, Isomil and Soyalac. By so doing, many potentially allergic infants may be fed soybean milk needlessly, but many allergists believe that this could possibly prevent or delay the onset of milk allergies in some babies. Other allergists believe soy milks can cause soybean allergies to develop in some children, and therefore recommend that these be tried only after an allergy to cow's milk develops.

One major disadvantage of soybean milk is its expense. Depending upon the baby's size, most infants would drink the contents of one or two cans each day. Soybean milk-fed babies grow as well as those fed cow's milk.

If cow's milk is to be given, it should be in the form of one of the lesser allergenic canned-milk types such as Similac. Milk proteins are changed by various heat treatments which make these types of milk less allergenic than fresh cow's milk.

### Is goat's milk less allergenic than cow's milk?

All milk can cause allergies, but whether it does or not depends upon which protein portion of the milk affects the child adversely. Sour milk separates into casein (the cottage cheese part) and whey (the clear liquid portion). Caseins of all animal milks are similar so that children allergic to cow casein would also probably be sensitive to goat casein. There are several proteins in whey which can cause allergy. It is possible on rare occasions to be allergic to a part of cow whey which is not exactly like goat whey. Such infants could drink goat's milk but would have symptoms from cow's milk. To complicate the interpretation, milk allergy can depend upon what the cow eats because the food proteins pass into the milk. A child may react to milk from cows fed moldy grain in the winter but not to milk from cows fed grass in the summer.

## Are there other milk substitutes for babies?

Yes. If your infant cannot tolerate soybean milk, which is in essence a bean soup, then various meat-soup "milks" can be tried. There are also predigested milk substitutes available such as Nutramigen but none of these should be used unless your physician gives you specific instructions. These milk substitutes are purchased at drugstores or large chain grocery stores. Corn, sugar or any additive in any canned milk can be a potential cause of allergy in some infants.

## Which cereals are least allergenic?

Once again the food causing allergy is more apt to be the one which is eaten most frequently. Rice, barley and oats all seem to be somewhat less allergenic than wheat and corn. An infant can become allergic to any cereal. Many allergists now recommend poi cereal of the type used in Hawaii. This, however, is not readily available in many localities. Rotate the cereals. Wheat on day one, oats on day two, barley or corn on day three, rice on day four.

## What are special toddler problems?

The major problem is the fact that they are walking or crawling and constantly playing in close contact with dusty floors. Carpets cause problems, even if synthetic, because it is impossible to keep them dust-free. Woolen carpets, of course, are especially bad since they also contain wool. Stuffed toys must be cotton inside and out. Toddlers often manage to get into substances which can cause allergic symptoms such as paint, hairspray, perfume or cleaning agents. Molds can be a problem.

## What should you do if your baby can't drink milk and won't drink soybean milk?

All growing children need calcium so that their bones will grow properly. If this is not supplied in the form of milk, soybean milk or dairy products, a calcium supplement must be taken. Infants can use a preparation such as Neo-Calglucon and older children can use DiCal-D wafers in the dose suggested by your physician. Watch to see if the mint flavor is a problem.

**Which soybean preparations are corn-free?**

Nursoy, Soyalac and 1–Soyalac. The last is not only corn-free, but lactose and milk-free.

**What causes the "terrible twos"?**

Children are normally very active around the age of two. Inquisitive, energetic children want to see and learn. Some allergists, however, believe that some of these children are abnormally overactive because of a sensitivity to food coloring and sugar, in particular. Other food suspects include milk, wheat, egg, corn, cocoa, preservatives, artificial flavors, peanut butter, orange, apple, grape and tomato. (See Chapter 9.) A one-week diet may give you the answer. Also try one Alka-Seltzer, *in gold foil* (without aspirin), and see if the overactivity stops in 15 minutes. If it does, the "terrible twos" may be due to a food sensitivity.

# CHAPTER 6

# *Hives*

**What are hives (urticaria)?**

These are itchy, red areas with white, raised, central circles which look like mosquito bites. They may come and go, for no apparent reason, over a period of one or two weeks. They are *always* initially caused by contact with something which has *never* caused trouble in the past. Unlike adults, who often have hives for months, children tend to have only one episode of hives without apparent cause.

A variant of hives is called angioedema—a marked swelling of the deeper skin tissues. It does not itch, although it may be painful.

Hives are made worse, regardless of the specific cause, by hot baths, overheating, exertion, pressure (as that from tight waist bands) or emotional upsets. Girls have hives more often than boys. We don't know why.

**How important is an occasional single hive?**

Usually it's not too important, unless it's very large or very itchy. If the hive has only a white, raised, central circular area and a circular ring of redness about it, it is probably caused by any number of things. If there is a tiny hole in the center of the central white area of the hive, it is probably due to an insect bite. By referring to the list of common substances causing hives (see below), you may be able to determine the cause of the problem without the help of a physician.

**What commonly causes hives or angioedema?**

Sudden hives and angioedema lasting a few days or weeks are most often due to the following, in this relative order: foods, drugs, miscellaneous substances and infection. An infrequent or unusual exposure often precipitates isolated attacks.

Chronic hives refer to those present for over a month. At times they recur for years. They are possibly due to drugs, infection and sometimes foods. Frequent or continued exposure to the same offending substance is more often the cause of the problem if it is prolonged.

## Which foods can cause hives?

| Most common | Others | |
|---|---|---|
| chocolate | alcohol (in medicines) | mint |
| eggs | beans | moldy foods |
| fish | cheese | mustard |
| fresh fruit | citrus fruits | pickles |
| (berries) | coloring (especially | pop (cola) |
| milk | red or purple) | preservatives |
| nuts | corn | (benzoic acid) |
| peas | gum | saccharin |
| pork | licorice | seasonings |
| shellfish | mayonnaise | spices |
| tomato products | meat sauces (soy) | vegetables (fresh) |
| | menthol | wheat |

## Which drugs can cause hives?

| Most common | Others |
|---|---|
| aspirin[1] | antibiotics (any type) |
| barbiturates | antihistamines |
| codeine | atropine |
| hormones as | chloral hydrate |
| ACTH | coal tar derivatives as |
| estrogens | acetanilide |
| insulin | antipyrine |
| pituitai y extract | digitalis |
| thiouracils or | dyes (candy, canned fruits, Jell-O, juices, |
| desiccated thyroid | margarine, medicines, vegetables, etc.) |
| penicillin[1,2] | eye, ear and nose drops |
| sulfonamides | heparin |
| | horse serum (antitoxins) |
| | iodides |
| | laxatives |
| | liver extract |
| | mercurials |
| | phenacetin |
| | phenolphthalein (laxatives) |
| | tonics |
| | toothpaste |
| | tranquilizers |
| | vitamins |

[1] These cause most drug allergies.
[2] Trace contaminants of this in milk, dairy products or chicken can sometimes cause prolonged chronic hives.

## Which infections can cause hives?

BACTERIAL—The tonsils, adenoids and teeth are the major areas but ears, sinuses, bladder or urinary tract and lungs can also be involved. Convalescence from scarlet fever or anthrax, brucellosis or pseudomonas infections also can be associated with hives.

VIRAL—It is noted with some viral infections, or after smallpox vaccinations.

FUNGAL—In association with infections of the feet or body.

SPIROCHETE—Especially after syphilis.

PARASITE—Any worm infestation or with Loeffler's disease.

PROTOZOAN—After malaria or Trichomonas infections.

## Which miscellaneous substances or diseases can cause hives?

| *Body preparations* | *Inhalants* | *Contactants* |
|---|---|---|
| body creams | aerosols | animal: dander, hair, saliva |
| body powders | ammonia | beetles |
| cosmetics | castor beans | butterflies |
| hair dye | cooking odors: | caterpillars |
| hair spray | eggs, fish | clothing dyes |
| mouthwash | flour | cocoons |
| nail polish | formaldehyde | feathers |
| soaps: bubble bath, | insecticides | foods[1] |
| perfume | paint | moths |
| toothpaste | sulfur dioxide | plants |
| wave set | tobacco | Portuguese man-of-war |
| | | silk |
| | | wool |

| *Allergens* | *Systemic diseases* | *Others* |
|---|---|---|
| castor beans | amyloidosis | chlorinated or water- |
| dust | infectious | softened water |
| excess allergy extract | mononucleosis | insect bites and scabies |
| dosage | kidney disease | mercury tooth fillings |
| molds or yeasts | leukemia | pregnancy |
| pets | liver disease | premenses |

[1] Any chemical such as insecticide, dye, wax or mold, in particular, on fresh fruits, vegetables or cheese.

| Allergens | Systemic diseases | Others |
|---|---|---|
| pollens | lupus erythematosus | dentures |
| stinging insects | malignancy | |
| | (Hodgkin's) | |
| | multiple myeloma | |
| | Raynaud's disease | |
| | rheumatoid disease | |
| | Stevens-Johnson | |
| | syndrome | |
| | thyrotoxicosis | |
| | ulcerative colitis | |

## How do you ascertain the exact cause of hives?

It is not easy. If you are not really interested in spending much time and effort, it is doubtful that the cause will be determined. The answer often lies in a detailed, hour-by-hour history of *everything* put into your child's mouth and any unusual contact for a full 24-hour period *prior* to the first hive or to a sudden onset of severe hives or swelling. At times hives appear immediately after the contact, but at other times it may be several or many hours before the itching is noted. If hives recur daily, something to which the child is often exposed is the cause. If the hives occur infrequently, something the child is seldom near or infrequently eats is the offender. At times it is the quantity of the allergenic substance which causes the difficulty. For example, eating a little chocolate almost daily may cause some children to have mild daily hives, but Easter time, with its bountiful supply, may precipitate severe hives and swelling. At other times it is the quality of the substance which is the offender. It may not be soup, but a certain brand of one special type. It may not be soda pop, but one certain flavor of a certain type. The records which are kept must be very specific and detailed.

If hives repeatedly occur, a study of records detailing events just prior to the onset of each episode is essential. It also helps if records are kept of the foods eaten, activities engaged in, and typical daily contacts for several 24-hour periods when no hives are noted. These would indicate which substances were probably not related to this problem and by comparing the records of so-called "good" 24-hour periods with "bad" 24-hour periods, the possible offending substances sometimes can easily be selected (see page 144 for more detail). Deliberate testing at some future time, *if the reaction is not severe,* or better, testing with your physician's help, will often confirm the exact cause of the hives. Sometimes the cause is never determined but the above method greatly increases the possibility of finding the answer to this difficult allergic problem. If you won't keep written records, the answer to your hives may remain elusive.

### How do you treat hives?

1. Apply, locally, calamine with phenol, which does not require a prescription.

2. Give an antihistamine such as Chewable Novahistine, for which no prescription is needed.

3. Give your child one Alka-Seltzer, *in gold foil,* if you feel a food caused the hives, unless the food was vomited immediately.

4. If the hives are very bad, an injection of long-acting epinephrine may be needed. This should be obtained from your physician or at the nearest hospital.

### What causes hives which occur during an infection?

It is frequently very difficult to determine exactly what is causing an episode of hives at this time. Any one of the drugs which a patient is receiving might be a factor, some infections can cause a hivelike rash, and it is also possible that a food which the child ate could be at fault. Under your physician's supervision, the usual procedure is to stop or replace most of the medicines which a child is receiving. (See Chapter 14.) If the hives stop in a few hours and do not recur, it is assumed that one of the drugs which was discontinued caused the problem. Unless the patient needed the suspected drug very badly, it would not ordinarily be given again to see if it was really the cause of the rash.

### What are the uncommon or rare causes of hives?

1. Heat, light or cold can cause them. Do not allow your child to swim in cold water if his hives are caused by cold, since a reaction to this could be very serious. If hives are caused by sunlight, use a sun-screening preparation, such as Uval. This problem often decreases after the child has a slight tan. Periactin helps cold urticaria.

2. There is a hereditary type of swelling without hives which occurs in certain families. The swelling does not pit, itch, hurt or look red. It may be associated with abdominal problems and occurs after trauma or near the menses in women. It can cause severe breathing problems and is due to the lack of an enzyme.

### Does skin testing help in the diagnosis of hives?

Hives usually occur only once and never again, so most children need treatment only for the initial episode. Children rarely have hives which last for long periods of time or recur often. Traditional skin tests are seldom helpful in finding the source of this type of problem, especially if the cause is a food. A detailed history can be more rewarding. Records of everything eaten or placed in the mouth and any unfamiliar contacts are more likely to reveal the cause. Skin tests may be helpful in diagnosing hives due to dust, pets, mold spores, pollens or stinging insects. Hives often prove to be a major challenge and the cause persists in being elusive and puzzling. Newer methods to skin test for foods, drugs, hormones, chemicals and other causes of allergy appear to be helpful in pinpointing definite causes of hives when other measures fail. (See Chapter 10 and Appendix V.)

### Does hyposensitization help hives?

Generally it is not indicated, but in a selected patient it might be helpful. This would depend upon the cause of the problem. It is possible to develop hives from grass, ragweed pollen, mold spores, stinging insects or dust, for example, and extract injections should help these patients. Newer methods to treat hives due to foods, in particular, show great promise although further scientific documentation is needed. (See Chapter 11.)

### What is dermographism?

Some children have skin which develops a linear or linelike hive if the skin is scratched by any pointed object, such as a fingernail. This does not indicate allergy. This is a trait often found in several members of a family.

### Are hives dangerous?

You may look terrible temporarily and feel unbelievably itchy, but hives are seldom dangerous. You need to be concerned, however, if the back of the throat swells or if your voice is becoming hoarse. Take an antihistamine and some asthma medicine (if these are available) and go directly to your physician or hospital. If a food could be the cause, take one teaspoon of baking soda in a glass of water.

### If you are desperate, what might help your hives?

Check with your physician first, but, sometimes, if you drink only spring water and eat carrots or possibly some honey for two days, the hives will go away. Put *nothing else* in your mouth, then add a single new food at every meal for several days. Sometimes this solves the problem quickly and inexpensively. Surprisingly, the food items which seem to cause hives at one time may not cause difficulty several weeks or months later. If you prefer, you can eat only the foods listed below for one full week. (See p. 166, *Rotary Diet*, and Chapter 9 for additional information.)

These foods are *least* apt to cause hives:

| | | |
|---|---|---|
| lamb | carrots | herb tea |
| rice | squash | spring water |
| barley | sweet potatoes | |

# CHAPTER 7

# *Unsuspected possible allergic diseases*

**What unrecognized signs and symptoms might be due to allergy?**
Some allergists and most ecologists believe the following chronic complaints can be caused by dust, pollen, pets, mold, food or chemical sensitivities. Many affected patients also have the more typical allergies, such as year-round hay fever or asthma, in themselves or their close relatives. The patients who do not recognize any clue indicating allergy in their family may never realize that their "learn to live with" complaints might be relieved by a simple change in their home or diet.

The major symptoms which a patient notices include headaches and muscle or joint aches. Children and adults often have leg pains which are unrelated to growing or exercise. Women often hold their shoulders high and have pain and tightness in the lower neck or upper shoulder area. Common intestinal complaints include recurrent abdominal pain, intermittent or daily diarrhea, constipation, nausea, and flatulence or belching. The abdomen suddenly may appear distended, particularly after eating an offending food. Halitosis, in spite of proper dental care, may be a chronic problem. This is often due to a milk, egg or wheat sensitivity. Some patients have sudden unexplained weight gain which seems to be due to fluid retention.

After eating allergenic foods for dinner, it is not uncommon to find that the next morning your fingers are too fat for the rings ordinarily worn. Canker sores or ulcers on the gums or inner lips are common, as is a mottled tongue with bald patches scattered over the surface. Children with this problem may wet the bed until they are teenagers and the family history often indicates that one of the parents had similar problems. Some children rush to the bathroom so that they don't have accidents, or find they have to urinate more often than normal. Insomnia is another complaint. Young children may have difficulty falling asleep and have frequent nightmares. Adults find they awaken at 3:00 or 4:00 A.M. and cannot fall asleep again. Adults or children may complain of itchy skin although no rash is evident. Affected children may be exceedingly ticklish. Children and adults with food allergies tend to have tiny pimples scattered over their buttocks. (Scratch marks located only in the area around the anus indicate possible pinworms.)

The major symptoms which affect the nervous system range from extreme fatigue, depression and inability to stay awake to uncontrollable hyperactivity, agitation and maniacal behavior. Children and adults complain that they have periods when they feel spaced out, cannot concentrate or think; their heads feel ballooned. They find they cry for little or no reason. Young children may have temper tantrums and often bite younger siblings or parents. Older children may be suicidal. Affected adults may have restless legs which they wiggle up and down rapidly or may sit and sway sideways, staring into space. Some children and adults have an unusual sensitivity to normal sounds or an intense dislike or compulsive preference for common odors. Some affected persons are aggressive, hostile and belligerent and destroy or hurt without feeling or remorse. Many parents complain that affected children do not want to be touched and resist being held, cuddled, loved or kissed.

Many of the symptoms described above are included in the allergic-tension-fatigue-syndrome which was initially described by Dr. Frederick Speer of Kansas City, in 1954. Portions of this syndrome were described as early as 1930 by Dr. Rowe as "allergic toxemia" and in 1947 by Dr. Theron Randolph of Chicago as "allergic fatigue." Many children and adults have varying combinations of the symptoms just mentioned. The same individual may have uncontrollable fatigue at certain times during the day contrasted with uncontrollable hyperactivity at other times. Of course, there are many other medical problems which can cause the types of symptoms which have been described. If you have seen many physicians only to be assured that your child's (or your) problems are not "organic," see Chapters 8 and 9. You or your child may not have to learn to live with illness or feel that a psychological problem is present when one does not exist.

### Can you suspect allergy by looking at a person?

Some of the following are not only characteristic of persons who have classical nose, eye and skin allergies and asthma, but also of patients who have allergies affecting other portions of the body.

## EYES

Many parents have observed dark circles under the eyes of their children. These circles can appear blue, black or red. Affected patients often have deep eye wrinkles which follow the lower eyelid across the skin below the eye. The eyelids may appear swollen or puffy. The eyelashes may be long, silky and attractive. Some children have tiny white scales on the eyelashes. The area below the eyes may be puffy so that there are bags under the eyes. Sometimes there are two bags, one directly below the eye and another rounded bulge below the outer edge of the eye in the region of the upper cheek. The eye circles (black eyes) and puffiness (bags under eyes) come and go depending upon the amount of exposure to allergenic substances. Many parents have commented that, when their child reacts to a food or a chemical, they notice a peculiar glassy look to the eyes just before and during the period of unusual activity or behavior. The face also may appear to have less expression than usual at that time. Watery, itchy, red eyes are classical symptoms of typical eye allergy.

## NOSE

Patients with typical nose allergy may have stuffiness or watery, runny nasal secretions. Because the nose is itchy, it is rubbed upwards, causing a horizontal wrinkle about ½ inch above the tip of the nose. This is often outlined with blackheads in adolescent children. Look in the mirror and push the tip of your nose upward toward the ceiling. Do you have a permanent wrinkle on your nose?

## EARLOBES

If your child's earlobes tend sporadically to become extremely red and warm, be suspicious of what was eaten shortly before.

## CHEEKS

It is not unusual for a small child's cheeks suddenly to look like two red, round, rouge patches shortly after exposure to an offending food or chemical.

## LIPS AND MOUTH AREA

The lips of allergic persons are often swollen and puffy. This may be an intermittent or a daily problem. The edges of the lips tend to be swollen, not sharp, and somewhat yellowish in color. The lips may show evidence of being chewed or bitten. Cracks in the corners of the mouth or central lip which do not respond to Vitamin $B_2$ also can be related to food sensitivities. Infants or small children with allergies may drool excessively, while older children and adults tend to lick their lips or the area about the mouth so frequently that a rash develops. Women who have pimples about their mouths and especially in the chin region (perioral dermatitis) often have a food sensitivity. Chocolate seems to be a common offender. A similar rash in children may be caused by contact with bubble gum, toothpaste, or a food, such as half an orange.

## FACE

Although this is not common, some children with allergy have very pale faces. Parents often believe them to be anemic. Once their allergy problems are resolved, their color improves markedly.

## VOICE

Children and women with allergy may have unusually high pitched, almost squeaky, voices which tend to become lower in tone when the offending item is avoided. Some stuttering, unclear speech and chronic laryngitis can be on a similar basis.

Hyperactive children tend to speak much and say little. After therapy they often continue to like to talk, but what they say has more meaning.

## HANDS

Stiff, swollen fingers in the morning may indicate early arthralgia, edema or fluid accumulation related to foods or chemicals. Persons with this problem often notice extreme weight gains of eight pounds or so within one or two days. In females, the menses may tend to cause unusual monthly weight gains which do not subside quickly.

The palms of children who have eczema may be extremely wrinkled.

## BODY

Some persons with body allergy have exquisitely tender skin spots which tend to come and go. These may be deep, localized areas of body swelling. The skin areas appear entirely normal except for the extreme tenderness.

Many children and adults seem to perspire excessively and some even have an unusual body or hair odor which is not eliminated with soap and water. This aroma may suddenly appear and disappear when a person is having a reaction to a food or chemical.

**What common unsuspected medical problems are possibly allergic in nature?**

Although stringent scientific documentation is not available at present, promising preliminary research indicates that *some* patients with the following chronic complaints have been helped significantly if the cause of their medical problem can be determined and eliminated. Once the offending foods, chemicals and contacts are avoided, it is not unusual for drug therapy to be reduced or discontinued.

## BLOOD VESSEL AND HEART DISEASE

Dr. William Rea of Dallas, Texas, has extensively studied many patients with a wide variety of blood vessel diseases. He has found that some patients who have rapid or irregular heart rates, high blood pressure, angina, thrombophlebitis (blood clots in legs) and coronary blood vessel spasm can be helped. He has scientifically documented that he can precipitate these medical problems by the ingestion of foods or exposures to common chemicals. Such patients are helped by avoiding the known chemical offenders and taking food therapy as outlined in Appendix VI.

## OBESITY

Although there are no large studies, there appears to be some evidence that obese persons crave foods, particularly wheat (flour) products, sugar and corn. These food cravings can be due to an allergy to these foods and, once the offending foods are avoided and the patient is treated, the craving can diminish along with the weight.

## NARCOLEPSY

This can be caused by a sensitivity to the exhaust fumes or the odors associated with new car upholstery, undercoating, carpeting or plastics. Some people become so sleepy that they cannot drive a car. An affected child may become so overcome by fatigue that his head will suddenly drop and hit the table during a meal. A mother may complain that she finds her child, who does not normally nap, asleep on the floor. She is alarmed because he cannot be awakened. Some adults find their muscles suddenly cannot support their weight and they fall to the floor, unable to arise for a while. Specific food and chemical exposures can cause these types of problems in some patients.

## ALCOHOLISM

Alcoholics often have a grain sensitivity to wheat, corn, rye or rice. Malt, sugar, yeast and grape also may be a problem. If a patient can drink Michelob beer but not other brands, a corn sensitivity, for example, may be present. It is of interest that persons who have this type of sensitivity often drink very little before they appear to be drunk. If they eat the food to which they are sensitive on an empty stomach, when they are *not* drinking, they may develop the identical symptoms which too much alcohol causes. Their favorite alcoholic beverage contains the food items to which they are sensitive.

## PSYCHOSIS AND NEUROSIS

Innumerable food and chemical exposures can produce different forms of neurotic and psychotic behavior. Good scientific documentation is now available for those who are interested. Movies and films which are anecdotal or single- and double-blinded are available through several ecologists. These problems are seen weekly in any busy ecologist's office.

## SEIZURES

There is documented proof that seizures have been precipitated in controlled hospital settings by the ingestion of foods or exposure to chemical odors. Abnormal electroencephalograms may return to normal after treatment or avoidance of known offenders.

## RENAL OR BLADDER DISEASE

Preliminary studies by Dr. Douglas Sandberg, in Miami Beach, Florida, have documented that nephrotic episodes can be precipitated by the ingestion of milk in some children. Avoidance or specific food therapy can prevent these episodes.

Enuresis or bed wetting, bloody urine, pain with urination, and the frequent need to urinate at times have been associated with food, chemical or pollen exposures.

## VERTIGO

In some patients, physicians have found that dizziness or ringing in the ears can be due to foods or chemicals.

## AUTISM

Recent preliminary studies by Dr. Dan O'Banion, of San Antonio, Texas, have shown that the ingestion of specific foods, after a period of fasting, can repeatedly cause changes in behavior and activity in autistic children. The same food can cause the same symptoms within the same period of time when the patient is repeatedly challenged.

## ULCERS, COLITIS, CROHN'S DISEASE

Dr. Albert Rowe described the favorable response of these medical problems to dietary management as early as 1930. More recent studies by Dr. Jacob Siegel, in Houston, Texas, have tended to confirm Rowe's original findings. Some ecologists claim success with various types of food therapy for chronic intestinal problems.

## FEMALE PROBLEMS

Very preliminary research conducted mainly by Dr. Richard Mabray, in Victoria, Texas, has shown that some patients with menstrual problems, breast tenderness, cystic breasts, extreme premenstrual tension, headaches, depression, chronic yeast infections and even endometriosis may have hormonal imbalances which sometimes respond quickly to the proper dilutions of progesterone or estrogen. Foods and chemicals may be associated problems.

## ARTHRITIS

More and more reports from several ecology hospital units indicate that some arthritic children and adults are being helped. It is possible to relieve some patients' symptoms greatly within a few days after fasting and to precipitate a recurrence of the joint problems within a few hours after the ingestion of offending foods. Arthritis caused by a single food exposure can last for several days. In the next few years, documented research to confirm these observations should be available.

## MULTIPLE SCLEROSIS, LUPUS ERYTHEMATOSUS

Although the data is scanty and inconclusive at present, there are early reports that these medical problems may be related to sensitivities to various environmental or food exposures. Favorable responses to therapy have been observed. No long-term follow-up is available at present.

## BEHAVIOR PROBLEMS

Barbara Reed, a probation officer in Cuyahoga Falls, Ohio, and A. Strauss and C. Simonsen, of City College, Seattle, Washington, have successfully helped chronic juvenile and adult offenders with diet therapy. They found that some of these individuals ingested excess amounts of "junk food," sugar and milk. When their diets were altered and the offending foods no longer consumed, the patients had a feeling of well-being and were able to work and function in an acceptable manner.

**What are the usual causes of unsuspected allergies?**

Major food offenders include milk, corn, wheat, egg, cocoa, sugar, coffee, food coloring, additives, preservatives, orange, grape, apple, tomato, pork, peanuts and cinnamon.

Common offending chemicals include tobacco, perfume, phenol, natural gas, gasoline, chlorine, synthetic household fibers such as polyester or polyurethane insulation material, soft plastic, insecticides, aerosols, auto exhaust and air pollution. Pollens, molds, pets and dust are also all significant factors in some patients.

The above common causes of traditional allergies such as year-round hay fever and asthma also cause allergy in less commonly recognized body areas. There is no reason medically to restrict allergy to arbitrary body areas such as the eyes, nose, lungs, skin and digestive tract. It appears that select areas of the brain, ears, throat, muscles, joints, bladder, vascular system and kidneys can be affected. In time, we also may find that the liver, spleen, specific blood cells, pancreas, thyroid, oviducts or any other body area can be affected.

**How can unsuspected allergies be diagnosed?**

There are a number of things which can be done safely and inexpensively to give some specific answers quickly.

1. Try the *Multiple Elimination Diet* in Chapter 9. Soon, one or more chronic symptoms may subside. When the individual foods are again eaten during the second part of the diet, it is possible to see quickly which food is causing symptoms.

2. Notice if symptoms subside when you travel, visit, camp, go into a hospital or are away from home. Are you worse when you return home? If the answer is yes, try to make your home more allergy-free as suggested in Chapter 8.

3. Try to test yourself for chemical sensitivities as suggested on pages 131–133. Don't, however, do these tests without close medical supervision if your reactions are alarming or frightening (for example, asthma, seizures).

4. If you suspect pollen, molds, dust or pets, find a physician who can do and properly interpret allergy skin tests or have an RAST study performed (p. 185) on your blood. These tests provide fast, accurate answers for many allergenic items but fail to detect many food and most chemical sensitivities.

5. Try Alka-Seltzer Antacid Formula without aspirin, in gold foil. If the symptoms subside within 20 minutes, be suspicious of a food which was ingested shortly before the appearance of the symptoms.

### How can undiagnosed allergy be treated?

It depends upon the cause.

If the cause is within your home, eliminate it or move to a house which does not contain that offending item. Live in your "new" home, however, for a while before you purchase it. It may contain other unsuspected offending items. People who move into new, modern, synthetic trailers are often disappointed to find that outgassing chemical odors continue to aggravate their medical problems.

If the cause is your diet, alter what you eat. If the food can be easily avoided—for example, banana, peanut, grape, orange or sugar—do not eat it. It requires much more determination and perseverance to avoid milk, wheat and egg in all forms. It is almost impossible to avoid corn, soy or all grains.

If you seem to have reactions to almost all foods, try the Rotary Diet on pages 166 to 175. This form of eating will quickly show you which foods you can tolerate and which you simply must stop eating. On a prolonged basis, this type of diet is thought to decrease the tendency to develop new food sensitivities.

Patients with severe food allergy sometimes are greatly relieved after fasting under close medical supervision in select hospitals directed by physicians knowledgeable about this form of allergy.

If the cause of an allergy is pollen, dust or molds, try these measures. If avoidance, cleaning and air purification are not effective, appropriate immunotherapy, as outlined on pages 187 to 199, may help relieve the symptoms.

If the cause is a chemical or due to air or water pollution, the challenge is immense. Special books, such as the recent one by Natalie Golos (page 328), give lists of unsuspected sources of contamination. To make the changes necessary to clean our air, water and soil will require a drastic change in the priorities of our government, with associated tremendous economic repercussions. There is no easy answer for many severely ill people. There are fewer and fewer "clean" places to hide and live.

## How can sudden unusual allergic symptoms be relieved?

A few suggestions might be helpful.

1. If you can remove yourself from the offending item, do so. If it is an odor, quickly get into the fresh air. Oxygen can be most beneficial. A hospital emergency room could supply this at the rate of about three to four liters per minute for a half hour or so.

2. If the cause is a food, try to vomit. Put your finger down your throat or use ipecac syrup which can be obtained from your pharmacist. A hospital emergency room might, under some conditions, have to pump out a patient's stomach.

3. If there is little available to relieve the situation, try ½ to one teaspoon baking soda in water.

If the problem is severe, intravenous sodium bicarbonate is sometimes most helpful and this can be obtained at hospital emergency rooms. For example, severe, sudden psychotic reactions at times can be relieved within ten minutes with this form of therapy. Due to the newness of this form of therapy, however, many physicians would not recognize or be knowledgeable about this form of medical relief.

## Can drug therapy be avoided with proper therapy?

Sometimes it can. When the nail is removed from the shoe, the sore heals. If the cause of hyperactivity is found, no Ritalin is needed. If the cause of gastrointestinal allergy is eliminated, no antacids are required. If the cause of a cardiac arrhythmia is found, no heart medicine may be necessary. If the cause of fluid retention is found, no diuretics are needed. If the cause of nose allergies is eliminated, no antihistamines are needed. Asthmatics can remain a tremendous medical challenge, although their need for medications often can be reduced when causative factors are eliminated.

Do *not* assume that all patients with these problems are helped so much that further medical supervision is not required. Many, however, appear to be aided to a gratifying and surprising degree.


# HYPERACTIVITY


## How can parents tell if their child is hyperactive?

A child can be hyperactive as a fetus. Mothers describe some hyperactive children as punching their way out of the uterus. As an infant, such a child may sleep little, cry often and immediately begin to stress the family unit. A hyperactive toddler may bump into so many walls and pieces of furniture that the parents are accused of battering. By school age, the hyperactive child is readily noticeable in a class of children. The nursery teacher can recognize the need for help very quickly.

A hyperactive child may not be able to join in games, listen to a story, sit through a meal or sleep through the night. Many cannot complete a chore, follow directions or accept correction or discipline. Due to problems in behavior and concentration, they often cannot learn effectively. They may be unable to adjust to siblings and parents at home, to classmates at school and to other children in the neighborhood. Their activities often lack direction or purpose.

**Are there different types of hyperactive children?**

Yes. There are happy and hostile hyperactive children. The happy ones are often humorous and entertaining, and giggle for hours during their whirls of aimless activity. The hostile ones tend to be mean and bite siblings, parents and friends. They are often unhappy, loud and disrespectful. Their behavior is often explosive. Discipline and reprimands during an acute reaction are useless.

When either of these types of hyperactive children are not adversely affected by foods and chemicals or pollens, they may appear and act entirely normal.

**How long do hyperactive periods last?**

It varies. The episodes can occur from within seconds to several hours (eight to sixteen) after the offending exposure and last from 20 minutes to a day or two. In general, however, most bouts of hyperactivity occur within a half hour and subside within two to four hours. The intensity and duration vary with innumerable factors. The most dramatic sustained reactions occur after a large quantity of an offending food is eaten on an empty stomach, when there has been no contact with the food in any form for about five to 12 days. Eating a small amount of an offending food in conjunction with other foods on a daily basis may mask symptoms and delude a patient into believing that a suspect food is not a problem.

**Can appropriate therapy improve a child's ability to learn?**

Maybe. Studies in the past ten years have shown that some children's I.Q.'s have increased after home and dietary changes, and allergy injection therapy. Some children labeled as MBD (minimally brain dysfunctioned) can show dramatic improvement. A double-blind study by Dr. James O'Shea in Lawrence, Massachusetts, in 1979, found food therapy was effective and children of varying intellects showed improvement in their ability to learn.

## Do hyperactive children need special guidance?

They often do. If a hyperactive child's problem is not resolved prior to school, multiple difficulties arise. The child's self image and worth are gradually abraded in the eyes of the child and his associates. Chronic home, school and friend problems cannot be solved by a "clean" bedroom, a special diet or food therapy. Personal and family psychological and social counseling may be essential.

## Are hyperactive adolescents special problems?

Yes. Nature seems to be on the side of adolescents in that in time they often tend to become less active or direct their activity along productive channels. In my experience, however, the teenager who has not been allowed to attend school for months or years due to unacceptable behavior and activity is a special challenge. Even when you have resolved the hyperactivity and behavior problems, the child will often refuse to accept the regimentation in school. They have lost their desire to catch up. How to help these young adults get back into the main stream of life is a major challenge. Many with the capability and desire to attend college will never realize that ambition. Counseling is often refused because, when it was tried *prior* to resolving the food or diet problem, it was not effective. When the youngster is calm and able to control and understand his activity and behavior, the same guidance which failed before might be successful.

## When can activity-modifying drugs be discontinued?

Older children or parents readily can tell when the drugs which control activity can be discontinued. Many can stop all drugs by the end of the first week of the diet. If the child seems more quiet, merely delay the next dose and see when it is needed. If it is, give it. If the child remains calm without the drug, it may not be needed. One young man who needed 180 mg. of Ritalin a day for ten years was able to discontinue the drug entirely after two days on the diet because he felt greatly improved as soon as food coloring and corn were eliminated.

Some children find that although they continue to need drugs to control their activity, when the drugs are combined with the diet, the control is much better.

### Will the teacher recognize your child's improvement?

If a child responds favorably, the vast majority of teachers can detect improvement in a child's activity and behavior within a few days. Most teachers are cooperative and anxious to help in every possible way. Occasionally, however, a child has been such a thorny, disruptive aggravation that a teacher may continue to overreact to the slightest provocation, even though there is definite evidence of improvement at home and in the neighborhood. In that situation, a new teacher in the same or a different school may be the answer.

### Why is there controversy about the cause of hyperactivity?

There are many reasons, one being that hyperactivity can be caused by many unrelated factors, some of them totally unrelated to food sensitivity or allergy. Physicians should remain skeptical until the medical literature supports a new viewpoint. Unfortunately, there are few double-blind reports *published* in accepted medical journals. Although diets *appear* to help, according to practicing physicians, parents, teachers and older children, long-term scientific studies need to be conducted. Medical journals are reluctant to publish articles by physicians in practice, even if they are double-blinded and documented with movies.

Most of the acceptable scientific studies which have been published to date have only suggested that there may be a relation between food coloring and activity. Unfortunately, in some of these studies all children were fed two identical types of cookies. One type contained food coloring and the other did not. It has been learned recently that there was not adequate food coloring in the one set of cookies to affect children who were sensitive to food coloring. In addition, *both* sets of cookies contained other foods, such as sugar, milk, wheat, egg and cocoa, which so often have been associated with heightened activity.

It may be possible that studies subsidized in part or wholly by the food industry may not be as impartial or unbiased as is necessary for valid scientific answers.

# PART THREE

# *How you can try to detect the cause of your allergies*

ALLERGIES sometimes can be relieved entirely or in part within one to two weeks by making changes inside a person's home or by altering what is eaten.

Chapter 8 helps you decide which type of home might be best and where it should be located. It details how to find out what is causing an allergy inside a house, room by room, item by item. It discusses the dry house, the damp house, problems from heating systems and the present-day interpretation of the value of air-conditioners and one type of air purifier.

If something in the home is contributing to an allergy problem, the simple changes recommended in this chapter often relieve symptoms within two weeks. These changes are sensible and practical. The bedroom must become an allergy-free oasis.

Chapter 9 explains how you may be able to determine which type of diet might help certain allergies. Foods which frequently cause allergic reactions are detailed. Common problems, pitfalls and dangers of diet studies are discussed. One note of caution: you should check with your physician before you embark on any diet.

# CHAPTER 8

# Allergies related to the home

**How can you select an allergy-free home?**

LOCATION—Pick an area that is dry and high. Don't move into an area with many trees, fields or factories, unless the prevailing winds tend to blow *away* from your home. Very windy areas should be avoided. Rural or suburban areas cause more pollen allergies than urban living. The latter, however, is often compromised by industrial or chemical pollution, *e.g.*, automobile exhaust fumes.

Don't pick a home in a heavily air-polluted area, such as one near an expressway, industrial area, granary, stables, gasoline stations, dumps or mills. Check with the local health department about the areas of town which are the least and most heavily polluted. At times, so-called "better areas" are surprisingly more highly polluted than middle class or poorer sections of cities.

Before a home is purchased, always check the basement to be certain there is no water level mark indicating previous flooding. If the soil near the home is so shaded and moist that grass won't grow, the home is apt to be musty or moldy.

AGE OF HOME—Extremely old homes can seldom be made allergy-free. Very new homes sometimes are irritating to the allergic child because of plaster dust, but are definitely preferable to old ones. Remodeling homes often precipitates allergy because of the accompanying increase in dust from plaster, wood, etc.

INSIDE THE HOME—Be certain it is not musty. Mustiness means that molds or fungi are present. To test for molds, you can obtain some Sabaraud's agar (it looks like tan Jell-O) in a round, flat, covered dish from the nearest hospital's bacteriology laboratory or from your physician. Keep the plates sealed and refrigerated until they are opened. Be sure to label each plate with your name, and the date and the room where it was opened. Merely open each plate for ten minutes in the room to be tested, then close it and seal it with Scotch tape. Return it to your allergist or bacteriologist within three days of exposure. Keep it meanwhile in a paper bag at room temperature. Most rooms should have only a few isolated colonies of growth on the agar.

Be certain the home is not drafty. If it is, seal the windows with cord or other caulking material obtainable at hardware stores, and use weather-stripping around the doors. The cord-caulking material can be removed easily in spring and replaced when cold weather begins.

Be sure that the people who previously lived in the house did not raise animals or do something which could cause problems long after you have moved in.[1]

### Is making your home allergy-free really important?

Yes. If your child has year-round symptoms, it is definitely essential. If a child has only seasonal problems when pollens are in the air, it is wise to make the bedroom allergy-free. The child who initially has only seasonal allergies often becomes allergic to winter allergenic substances in a few years' time.

These precautions also may help to prevent any other children, who do not have allergic symptoms, from developing them in the future. The more of these recommendations you follow, the sooner your allergic child should improve. Parents who make excuses, valid or otherwise, have children who take longer before they respond favorably to therapy.

### How can you tell if something in your home is causing your child's allergy?

A clue may be provided if you find that your child is very well whenever he is in the hospital but immediately becomes ill after a short period of time at home. Such children are often healthy when the family is camping or on vacation; this also points to a problem within the home. If you believe your home is at fault and do not want to leave town, arrange to camp outside, rent a motel room or stay with relatives or friends for a few days. Then, if your child sleeps well at night and requires no medication, there probably is something in your home causing the allergy.

Beware, however, of taking household goods, such as pillows, if you want to determine if your child is better away from home. The items you carry may be the part of your home causing the difficulty. Foods are not a factor if your child is better when not living at home, provided that your child's diet remains essentially the same.

---

[1] Fumigation or urethane blown into the walls for insulation could cause prolonged home pollution.

**How can you tell that a certain room is causing allergies?**

Watch your child. Do the symptoms occur mainly in the kitchen or bathroom, during the night, or the first thing in the morning? This means that the room the child was in, just before symptoms occurred, probably contains the offending substances or odors. Any sudden change, coughing spell or series of sneezes should alert you. If your child is playing with a certain toy or sitting in a specific place whenever the symptoms occur, the cause of the symptoms may lie there. It could be related to the inside or outside of a toy or to the covering or stuffing of furniture in the vicinity. Draperies, carpets, wallpaper, insulation, heating fuel or a cleaning agent or odors may be at fault.

## BEDROOM

**Why is the bedroom so important in relation to allergies?**

There are two major reasons:

1. This is the room where your child spends more time during a 24-hour period than in any other room. If your child breathes "pure" air for eight to ten hours each night, he can tolerate more exposure to allergenic substances during the daytime. Most children have more allergy symptoms at night than during the daytime, so keeping this room allergy-free is essential. Lying flat all night frequently stuffs the child's nose and allows mucous secretions in the lung to possibly collect or pool in certain areas which can trigger coughing episodes and possibly wheezing.

2. It is impossible for a busy housewife to keep her whole home allergy-free. By making the bedroom so, it is easier for her to clean it and to keep this as a haven for her child. Allergic persons need an allergy-free oasis in their home.

**How do you make a bedroom allergy-free?**

This is the room where you spend a major portion of each day. Strip the room and make it look like an army barracks, no clutter, everything in drawers or in an enclosed metal or wooden bookcase.

*Bedding:* Use 100 per cent cotton, free of chemical finishes, polyester and odor retardants, for sheets, pillowcases, mattress pads and blankets. A drop of water should immediately soak in to an untreated fabric. Don't use an electric blanket. The odor of the heated plastic wires can cause symptoms in some patients. The pillow should be soft, untreated cotton. Stuff an untreated cotton pillowcase with cotton blanketing, cotton towels or cotton batting. The use of feather or down pillows can predispose you to a feather sensitivity. Most new down pillows are chemically treated. Also, avoid polyurethane, Dacron, Acrylon, foam rubber, kapok and hair-filled pillows.

*Mattresses:* Try a canvas-mattress cot or sleep on a bare wooden floor temporarily until you decide if a change is needed. Special untreated 100 per cent cotton mattresses are available[1] with pure cotton-barrier cloth covers. Avoid sanitized mattresses with moldy odors, chemical finishes, flame or mold retardants, polyurethane or foam rubber. Old mattresses in good condition may be satisfactory if enclosed in a cotton-barrier cloth cover.

*Box springs:* Use a coiled type with an untreated cotton cover. Avoid foam rubber. Encase in a cotton-barrier cloth cover.

*Bed:* Avoid headboards with storage areas, ornate carving or vinyl trim. Canopy beds, bunk beds or underbed storage types can be dusty, thus contributing to symptoms.

*Furniture:* Wood (except pine) and metal are best. Naugahyde, odorous plastic or upholstered items with synthetic filling may cause symptoms. Keep the dresser tops bare, except for necessities, clock, radio, lamp. Store no items with odors in the dresser. Keep bookcases outside of the bedroom, if possible.

*Toys:* Keep toys in a metal or closed wooden box or bookcase. The toys should be entirely metal, wood or 100 per cent cotton. Avoid plastic. Toys filled with kapok, feathers, wool, rabbit fur and any odorous synthetic stuffing can potentially cause symptoms. If you burn a little of the stuffing and it smells like a singed chicken, it means that it contains animal hair. Replace the filling with untreated cotton.

*Walls:* Painted plaster walls, non-asbestos wall board, birch or oak panelling are best. Avoid pine or drywall. Walls can be painted with Sherwin-Williams Soy Alkyd (Duron) paint or Du Pont Lucite (*without* Teflon) or with casein-type paints. Add one box of baking soda to each gallon of latex, water-based paint to reduce odors emitted from fresh paint. If preferred, walls can be covered with vinyl, non-plastic or aluminum wallpaper (*without* Mylar). Prepasted wallpaper with fungicides is not advised. For paste, use wheat starch or Argo box starch with water and calcium proprionate as a mold-retardant. Remove old, flaking or moldy wallpaper. Allow no fabric-covered walls, pennants, pictures, chalkboards or dust-collecting, hanging decorations.

*Windows:* Untreated cotton curtains are best. Beware of odorous plasticized shades, venetian blinds, ruffles, polyester blends, straw curtains, corduroy, rough textures, fiberglass or hair blends.

*Floors:* The most practical floor is plain wood. If it must be covered,

[1] See Appendix IV, page 282.

use an old, untreated, cotton carpet or scatter rug. Some Sears, Roebuck indoor-outdoor, tight-weave, low-nap, non-odorous carpets with jute backing may be tolerated. Have the child sit directly on the carpet for at least half an hour prior to purchase. Notice if any symptoms occur. In some areas of the country, stone, terrazzo, smooth cement, brick, terra-cotta or ceramic tile are acceptable. Avoid asbestos tile, asphalt-based adhesives, plastic linoleum, hardwood finishes or waxes, synthetic, odorous carpeting, shag rugs or nylon carpets with hair (ozite), foam rubber, glue or plastic backing.

*Vacuuming:* A central vacuum cleaner with metal dusts is best. Water-type tanks (Rex Air) are next best, but hot motor oils can be offensive. Most upright vacuum cleaners leak dust, emit motor odors and may have chemically treated disposable bags.

*Closets:* Allow only the clothing which is presently being worn. The odor of mothballs, insect repellent strips, plastic garment or cleaning bags or cedar can be offensive. Chemical odors from freshly dry-cleaned clothes can cause symptoms in some patients.

## LIVING ROOM

As in the bedroom, wood, metal, glass, cotton and Formica are best. Older genuine leather-covered furniture is expensive, but usually well tolerated. Avoid odorous furniture polish or carpet shampoos.

*Toss pillows* must be made of untreated cotton both inside and outside. They may have to be homemade.

*Flowers:* Artificial bouquets may have a chemical odor and tend to become dusty. If the flowers are fresh, pollen can be shaken from them as they are carried or arranged, causing symptoms. If they are not fresh, molds can be a problem. Any person sensitive to ragweed probably will have symptoms when exposed to marigolds or chrysanthemums. For *play area* for small children in front of the television, use an untreated cotton blanket or a sheet of oak or birch panelling.

*Pets:* All pets with hair or fur have dander. The hair and dander gradually accumulate and, even when the pet is not in the room, there may be enough hair and dander in the air, on walls, in heating ducts and on furniture to cause symptoms. When a pet is no longer in a home, symptoms can persist for weeks even though the pet-contaminated area has been meticulously cleaned.

## BATHROOM

The sink, toilet and tub should be porcelain in composition, not

plastic or synthetic. The shower stall must be tile, and not plasticized.
*Bathtub:* If chlorine is a problem, add a few crystals of sodium thio-sulfate to the bath water.
*Shower curtains:* Use no odorous plasticized fabrics or material. Un-finished, 100 per cent terry cloth is best.
*Shower stalls:* Use tile, not a plasticized substitute. Avoid synthetic glue. Sand and cement which are not quick-drying are tolerated.
*Toilet seats:* Use wood, never plasticized rubber cushioning.
*General:* Allow no scented items for cleaning or body care. Pleasant-smelling body lotions, underarm deodorants, hair spray, after-shave lotions, powders, creams, shampoos, toilet paper, facial tissues or cleaning aerosols often cannot be tolerated. Women can be sensitive to the chemicals in or on various items used for feminine hygiene. Internal, chemically treated tampons can be replaced with removable plugs of natural sponge if the former present a problem. Avoid the chemical odor of hair dyes or permanent wave preparations.

For tooth care, try a combination of sea salt (from the health food store) and baking soda. Toothpaste can contain dyes, flavors and sugar which can adversely affect some children, although some health food store varieties may be tolerated. The same is true for mouthwash or any pill or liquid medicine.

## KITCHEN

### What causes allergy in a kitchen?

The usual items are scented cleaning materials and carpets. Persons with chemical sensitivity must also consider the following:
*Stove:* Gas stove fumes can cause diverse complaints, particularly head-ache and joint pains. Use only an electric stove. Be sure there is ade-quate ventilation and an exhaust fan. Never heat canned foods directly upon a burner. The phenolic lining from the inside surfaces of cans can cause sensitivity.
*Refrigerator:* Purchase an electric, porcelain or steel, commercial, low-humidity refrigerator without a self-defrost and with a minimum of plastic-coated wire. Use baking soda to diminish inside odors. Wipe rubber parts with vinegar to retard mold growth. Use no plastic con-tainers, food bags or soft polyethylene covering. Store all left-over foods in glass, steel or ceramic containers, never in plastic.
*Cabinets* should be wood, metal or Formica.
*Floor:* Use Armstrong inlaid linoleum. Use no asphalt adhesive.
*Table tops:* Use Formica, old Bakelite, stainless steel or wood.

*Pots and pans:* Stainless steel, ceramic, Pyrex and cast iron are best. Avoid non-stick sprays and utensils, aluminum or plastic. Use no aerosol oven cleaners. Install Corningware chopping blocks.

*Ironing board pads:* Must be 100 per cent cotton.

*Dishwasher:* This should have a stainless-steel interior.

*Cleaning:* For the kitchen, use Borax or Rokeach Kosher Soap. Avoid all kitchen aerosols, floor wax or odoriferous cleaning agents such as scouring powder. Bon Ami cake soap is acceptable.

*For the laundry,* use Oakite. Miracle White is better than chlorine bleach because odor of the latter in the laundry (or pool) area can cause symptoms in some sensitive persons.

*Clothes washer and dryer:* Both must be electric. Dryer must be vented to the outside to reduce mold contamination.

## OTHER TIPS

*Clothing:* Gloves, slippers, muffs, hats or sweaters should not be trimmed with rabbit fur. Feather trimming must be avoided. One unsuspected source of mold is winter boots, which become damp, wet and moldy. Each time the child handles his shoes and socks, the mold comes in contact with his hands.

Chemically sensitive patients are sometimes affected by an odor from modern fabrics. Before wearing, soak them in a quarter tub of water after adding two cups of vinegar or Borax. It may be necessary to do this several times.

*Insects:* More and more evidence points to the fact that disintegrating dead insects of various types can cause allergies. These include sand flies, beetles, mites, cockroaches, and so forth. Every effort must be made to eliminate these from your home *without* using an insecticide, which in itself will cause symptoms. Vacuum furniture often and well to decrease mites in couches, chairs and mattresses. Beware of pest strips.

*Newspaper:* Newspapers can cause symptoms because of the ink or odor. Drying the paper in the oven sometimes helps. Some people are so sensitive that they have to read the paper inside a glass box. Certain dyed sections of the paper often have offensive chemical odors, as do some types of magazines or books.

*Insulation:* The chemical type (for example, urea formaldehyde foam) which is sprayed into the walls can cause devastating problems to persons sensitive to the odor. Yellow, not red, fiberglass may be tolerated if it is wrapped in aluminum, not chemically treated, paper.

*Appliances:* Try to purchase only electric-type hot-water heaters, stoves, clothes washers, dryers, etc.

*Lights:* Avoid fluorescent types because the ozone, radiation and limited spectrum of these lights have been associated with increased activity and irritability in some children and adults. Full-spectrum lighting with radiation shields is available, but quite expensive.

*Apartment Living:* Try to live above the fifth floor, the higher the better. Select an apartment which does not face a polluted area of the town or the street. Pollution maps and information about the prevailing winds can be obtained from the local health department. Do not live near the building's incinerator. Do not tolerate routine insect extermination. Insist on wooden floors rather than wall-to-wall carpeting.

*Telephone:* Some people are sensitive to the odor of plasticized phones or to the chemical-impregnated cotton located in the listening section of the receiver. Unscrew the cover and remove it.

## OUTDOORS

### What causes allergies in the immediate vicinity of your home?

GRASS—This can cause allergic symptoms when it is pollinating. Lawns have a whitish appearance when the grass is pollinating heavily. If the grass is cut short and often, before it pollinates, it causes fewer symptoms. Children should not play on recently cut lawns. Older grass-sensitive children can cut the lawn at certain times when there is relatively little grass pollen, but at other times can become quite ill with asthma or hay fever if grass pollen is abundant. Grass odors or terpines also cause symptoms.

In the early spring after the snow melts, molds can be found on the grass, which can cause potential difficulty. In the fall, and during damp periods, molds are again plentiful. Children who play ball on the grass frequently handle the grass molds and pollen.

Seeding lawns, using fertilizers and various lawn herbicides have been known to precipitate allergic symptoms.

LANDSCAPING—Most flowers do not cause allergic symptoms unless they are repeatedly held near the nose so that sensitization occurs. The major problems occur when attempts are made by allergic children to help remove weeds from home borders. Molds can contaminate plants and soil. Some garden sprays or insecticides seem to cause allergies.

TREES—These cause symptoms only in the spring when the flowers appear, usually just before the leaves are evident, and then again when the leaves fall. Trees which are located very close to the patient's bedroom can be a potential source of difficulty. Some trees with large or colorful flowers, such as chestnut or fruit trees, do not cause allergies because they are insect pollinated. Their pollen is mainly spread by insects and not by wind. Orchard growers often lament excess rain during the flowering period, for fruit will not develop when bees aren't active.

Attempts to rake leaves or to play in leaf piles can cause symptoms because of the molds, especially *Pullularia,* which are often found on the leaves.

AIR POLLUTION—Although a direct causal relationship between allergies and air pollution, other than with pollens, is not completely confirmed, research is presently being carried out to attempt to correlate such impressions. It is believed possible that some factory contaminants do directly or indirectly precipitate allergic symptoms, either immediately or several hours after exposure. Symptoms are also seemingly related to the community or large-scale use of insecticides over orchards, crops or insect-infested areas. An attempt should be made by parents to notice if certain odors, thermal inversions or atmospheric pollutants repeatedly seem to be related to their child's symptoms. Some health departments are very interested in such information.

Mass spraying for insects or fertilizing can precipitate asthma or other symptoms in chemically-sensitive patients.

## MOLDS

**How can one decrease the mold contamination in a home or basement?**

1. Remove as much of the mold-contaminated material as possible. Carpets or leather products, for example, are sometimes moldy. Check all foam-rubber products, even new ones, because these frequently become moldy if wet or stored in a damp place. Camping equipment, stored vegetables, fruits or grains, books and flowers are also often contaminated.

2. Install a dehumidifier. It is often amazing how much water will be eliminated each day.

3. For cleaning moldy areas, dilute one ounce of concentrated 17 per cent aqueous Zephiran chloride in one gallon of water. This can be purchased in a drugstore.

Borax is also helpful and can be used in the laundry to reduce the mold which grows quickly on soiled, damp clothing, or in wet towels or washclothes.

4. Use a mold-resistant paint. This can be obtained from Sherwin-Williams and is called Loxon. It is a latex, water-soluble paint for use in moldy basements. See Appendix IV, pp. 287–8.

# HOUSE DUST

## What exactly is house dust?

This is thought to be composed mainly of disintegrated fiber or cellulose material in houses. This would include broken-down cotton,
kapok or feather furniture stuffing, draperies or furniture coverings,
molds, food particles, insecticides, wool, mites and, in some homes,
animal hair or dander from pets or from carpet pads. Outside dirt or
clean sand does not usually cause allergies.

## What is an autogenous dust?

This is a special extract made from the dust collected in the vacuum
cleaner in your home. Usually about two full-packed quarts are needed
to prepare the extract and your allergist can send this to a laboratory.
Preparation requires about a month. Dust should be collected by vacuuming your child's bedroom and any other room which he frequently
uses. (Do not collect dust if carpet has just been chemically cleaned,
or at Christmas time, because pine needles would not ordinarily be a
part of your home's debris.)

## What is the advantage of an autogenous dust?

In rare cases the regular dust which your allergist uses does not help
a particular child. If a child does not respond well to the allergy treatments, special autogenous dust may be more effective. Dust in your
home contains the exact substances which your child is breathing and
treatment extracts derived from it should give the best protection. The
use of this type of dust is not necessary for most patients but occasionally, especially if there is anything unusual about a child's home,
it is essential. Some homes, for example, are very old, or filled with
antiques, or may contain Oriental carpets, pets, or something which
makes that particular house unique in its dust composition.

## Can you test to see if house dust causes allergy?

You can test your child but this could cause sudden, severe and
dangerous allergic symptoms. For this reason purposeful exposure
should be carried out only under an allergist's supervision. However,
if you notice that changing the vacuum cleaner bag or dusting with a
mop or cloth always causes allergies in your child, no further evidence
is needed.

## HEAT

### How important is the type of heat used in the home?

There is no easy practical answer. Some children may have no significant chemical problem *at the present time*. There are no studies to indicate how many children will develop chemical problems as they age. For years, a forced hot-air heating system with an air-conditioner and an air purifier was suggested for pollen and dust-sensitive patients. Many patients appear to improve, at least on a temporary basis, with either furnace or room units which purify and cool the air.

In our chemically contaminated world we must wonder if we should not strive to *prevent* future sensitization. Solar heat would be ideal but is still not practical. This leaves electric hot water heat or low temperature, electric baseboard heat from units stripped of all rubber or plastic parts. The latter units must be easy to vacuum. If hot water heat is used, it should not be dependent on gas or oil because fumes can often cause illness. If you have few choices, seal the register (if any) in the affected child's room with a double layer of heavy-duty aluminum foil attached with freezer-type tape. Then install an unpainted, low-temperature, electric, baseboard room heater free of plastic and rubber parts and an insulation-free air-conditioner ordered directly from the manufacturer. This should make this one room more chemically-free and comfortable.

Another possibility is hot water heat in copper coils or pipes in terrazzo floors.

If the furnace is circulating chemicals due to the use of fossil fuel (gas, oil and coal), some chemically-sensitive persons will remain ill. This problem can be reduced by installing the furnace in a separate building outside the home or by the use of an eductor fan in the chimney so that the blower draws combustion products from the furnace or boiler and expels them up the chimney.

### What problems are noted with a forced hot-air heating system?

This type of heat utilizes a blower to circulate the air. Unless supplementary humidification is supplied, this tends to be drying.

If your furnace does not have an electrostatic-precipitation unit, the furnace filters must be changed often. If this is not done, the efficiency of the furnace is diminished while the cost of heating your home is raised.

Most furnace filters should be changed at least monthly. There are two major types—throw-aways, which cost relatively little and are used for a month and then replaced, and the permanent type, which initially cost more but last for prolonged periods and can be washed as often as necessary. These, however, can become moldy.

If the furnace filters are not cleaned regularly, the ducts or conduits leading from the furnace to various rooms can become very dusty and dirty. Whenever the blower is on, this dust can be circulated through your home. You can check to see how much dust is being forced into various rooms by covering the heating outlet with a porous, coarse cloth such as muslin, cheesecloth, or a thin layer of fiberglass or glass floss. If the cloth is too thick it will noticeably diminish the heat in the room where it is being used. If the cloth is soiled repeatedly, it could indicate that the ducts need to be cleaned or, in rare cases, that your furnace needs to be examined for cracks. Although the efficiency of duct cleaning is not ideal, your furnace specialist should be able to advise you about who is most capable of doing such work. Immediately following cleaning, be certain to cover all registers with fiberglass or cloth because loose dust can be a problem for a few days.

## AUTOMOBILE

### How do automobiles cause allergies?

Some children have allergic symptoms whenever they ride in a car. This could be caused by dust, cigarette smoke or other air pollutants. Mold spores can be a problem if the car ever becomes damp or is accidentally left open during a rainstorm. If the windows of the car are open, any area which is passed could cause immediate symptoms. Examples would be fields of pollinating plants, factory or dump odors and grain mill pollution.

The odor of new cars can cause symptoms in some persons. In particular, the smell of plastic or vinyl trim, seats and undercoating can be offensive. These odors may dissipate in time. Notice if anyone sniffles or develops a headache or behavior problems when the family is out for a drive.

In the winter, heaters often circulate dust and pollutants inside cars. In the summer, open air vents also circulate road dust and pollens.

Car air-conditioners sometimes help to diminish allergic symptoms. If the outside air vents are kept closed so that the air within the car is continually being recirculated, this helps to diminish the road dust and pollen which can enter the car. Car air-conditioners contain evaporator coils which supposedly trap small amounts of smoke and pollen particles as they condense moisture. Their major function, however, is to cool the air and remove moisture from it.

## HUMIDITY

### Is humidity a factor related to allergies?

Yes. The mucous membranes or tissues which line your child's nose and lungs must be moist so that the tiny hairs which surround this breathing passageway can move a thin film of mucus towards the throat. If the membranes become dry, the hairs which help to keep the breathing tubes clean cannot function properly. This leads in turn to respiratory problems and could also make a child more prone to infection.

Humidity varies with the type of home and the time of year. Most homes are too dry in winter and therefore require a humidifier. These same homes are too damp in the spring and summer and need a dehumidifier.

Dust also settles in rooms where the humidity is normal, but tends to remain in the air if the atmosphere is very dry. Vaporizers should be used if they seem to help. If you are unsure about them or if the child or infant becomes worse under their influence, do not use them. There is some evidence that cool-moisture vaporizers seem to be more helpful than warm-mist vaporizers. The latter, however, would tend to thin mucus so that it could be coughed up more readily. Use whichever seems to help your youngster most. Always be certain to clean vaporizers or room humidifiers thoroughly with aqueous Zephiran, because these machines can spread infection if they are contaminated. Do not use irritating or odorous chemical solutions for cleaning.

### What is relative humidity?

This is the amount of moisture in the air compared to the amount of moisture the air can actually hold at a given temperature.

### What is the usual winter-time relative humidity in the average home in a cold area of the United States?

It would vary from about 12 to 20 per cent. A desert has a relative humidity of about 25 per cent.

### What should the humidity in your home be?

Ideally, about 40 or 50 per cent with an indoor temperature of 68° or 70° F. (20°–21° C.). However, if the outside temperature is about 0° F. (−18° C.), a home relative humidity of 25 per cent is recommended. If the outside temperature is 20° F. (−7° C.) or above, inside it should be about 35 per cent. Lower than average room temperatures are more tolerable if humidification is adequate.

**How do you measure the relative humidity?**

A device called a Humidiguide, obtainable at many hardware stores, will measure relative humidity. It is easier to read than a body thermometer.

Each room should be checked because there may be some variation among different rooms of the same house. This problem can be resolved if free circulation of air is permitted by keeping the inside doors open. Attempts should be made to adjust humidity toward normal levels.

**What is the optimal temperature for an allergic child's room?**

There is no clear-cut answer. If a room is too hot or cold, it can contribute to a child's problems, just as any rapid change in temperature does. Generally, the bedroom temperature should not fall below 68° F. (20° C.). Children should be discouraged from walking on cold bedroom floors without slippers. Foot pajamas or bed socks can help to prevent this problem.

## AIR CLEANERS

**What is an air cleaner?**

This is a machine which cleans the air as it is circulated within a room. Most air purifiers clean by means of filters which sift out large and small particles; others clean by electronically precipitating the air particles onto charged collection plates which are washed at regular intervals. These air cleaners are helpful if pollen, dust, molds, smoke, etc., are major problems causing allergy. Some patients improve within 24 hours.

Some, however, are not only not helpful, but can also be harmful for persons who have chemical-type allergies. Some HEPA filters produce offensive chemical odors due to glue and sealers, while room and furnace electrostatic units emit ozone and nitrous oxide, which some people find objectionable. Also, be wary of buying inexpensive or undersized units. Try to obtain the type you select on a trial basis with a money-back guarantee if it is unsatisfactory.

**Which air-depollution unit is best?**

If your aim is to clean the air and decrease chemical contamination, the unit suggested on page 127 is best. This unit not only removes the solid and gaseous chemical contaminants but it also does not *add* any additional chemical contaminants to the air emitted from the machine. To accomplish this purpose, these units not only utilize a particulate filter but also have a layer of activated alumina impregnated with potassium permanganate (Purifil) sandwiched between two separate sections of activated carbon. The latter are available as coconut, or bituminous or anthracite coal-based charcoal. These units have a high energy efficiency ratio (EER) of at least 10.

### Is a furnace electrostatic-precipitation unit or a room unit best?

Both have advantages and disadvantages. A room unit of proper size will usually keep a room so clean that no dust accumulates. It is about the size of a large typewriter and can easily be lifted by an adult. It helps a child, however, only while he is in the room that contains the air-cleaning unit.

A furnace unit may clean rooms unevenly, just as a furnace heats some rooms better than others. Truly balanced heat is often an ideal, not a reality. Furnace units, however, would diminish the total pollen and dust count in the whole house. Some furnace units are so effective that homes are truly dust-free. If several members of a family had allergies, this unit would be preferred. Furnace units can be used only in homes which have a forced hot-air heating system.

### Where should the electrostatic-precipitation unit be placed in a bedroom?

Do not have the machine face the child directly since it causes a draft of cool air. Have the air circulate in the direction of your child's feet. The machine can be placed on top of the dresser or on the floor, well away from the wall. Keep the doors and windows closed at all times.

### Are room units difficult to clean?

It would vary with the type of unit. To clean the portable Micronaire unit, for example, disconnect the machine from the electrical circuit and remove four thumbscrews from the back. Remove the central piece with the many charged plates and put the entire piece in detergent water or rinse in the sink using a hose. You will be surprised at the amount of dust which will come from the plates. The activated carbon filter, which decreases ozone emission in the Micronaire units, can be removed and cleaned separately. It must be replaced at regular intervals.

### Which air-conditioner unit is best?

Due to chemical odors from plastic wires and motor oils, special units must be ordered during the winter so that they will be available for use in summertime.

### Are furnace de-pollution units available?

A room de-pollution unit and air-conditioner are more efficient. For example, these units might make a room which is chemically contaminated with gas fumes tolerable for a person who could not afford electric heating. Electrical heating, however, is essential for anyone with an extreme natural gas sensitivity.

### Are there maintenance problems with air de-pollution units?

One merely has to replace the charcoal and Purifil filters every three months.

### What causes the characteristic odor noted with electrostatic-precipitation units?

This is caused by ozone. Ozone is a form of oxygen which has an extra atom of oxygen ($O_3$) and a peculiar characteristic odor. The amount of ozone which a machine produces usually diminishes after just a few days. If it does not, return the machine. Many people find a slight ozone odor refreshing. To a degree, this will vary with the amount of ozone the machine produces, and some produce more than others. An excess of ozone can be offensive, irritating to the respiratory tract, and *toxic*. Levels over 0.05 p.p.m. are undesirable. But there is no easy way to determine how much ozone a machine emits. Activated carbon filters decrease ozone emission.

The odors of heated plastic, oils or paint can be a problem for the chemically sensitive patient.

### How many hours should the machine be used each day?

It is recommended that most air-purifying units be used 24 hours a day in order to ensure maximum air purification. If the sound (a faint hum) is an annoyance, use it during the daytime only. Perhaps during the night it can be put in another room which the child frequently uses.

### Can an air-purifying machine be used if windows are left open?

Yes, but it would not work as effectively since it could not keep the air clean if the air is being continually changed. It certainly would remove some of the pollen or dust. Place the air purifier between the window and the child's bed. Direct the flow of air so that it indirectly bounces off the wall near the bed and then passes toward the child's face. This will eliminate a draft but allow the child to breathe relatively clean air. Children tend to leave doors open, so a spring should be attached to help keep the bedroom door closed.

**When would be the best time to air out a bedroom?**

Do it in midday, because in the early morning hours (4:00 to 8:00 A.M.) pollens are more prevalent. Pollen tends to be less of a problem at midday than at other times.

**Do furnace electrostatic-precipitation units function with uniform efficiency throughout the year?**

No. If you heat by hot air, the blower is normally utilized only when heat is being produced. The unit therefore is removing air impurities only when the blower is on and this would be intermittent, depending on how often the temperature drops low enough to trigger the heating mechanism to produce more hot air. Ideally, therefore, the blower should constantly be "on" if the air is to be cleaned as much as possible.

During the summer, if you have a furnace electrostatic-precipitation unit, the blower should be functioning constantly so that the air is continually being circulated and cleaned. If you do not have an air-conditioner, the house will become warm. If windows and outside doors are kept open, the efficiency of air-cleaning would be reduced. However, if the furnace unit were working constantly, it would remove at least part of the pollen and dust even if the windows were open.

## AIR-CONDITIONERS

**Do air-conditioners help allergies?**

While many children and adults find that their allergic symptoms clear immediately in an air-conditioned area, others instantly become worse even if exposed for a short period of time. The reason for this is not easily explained. Any sudden change in temperature, however, can cause allergic symptoms in some individuals. Check your child's response to an air-conditioner before investing in one.

**Do air-conditioners remove pollens?**

While air-cleaning units will remove over 90 per cent of the pollen granules and smaller particles, such as smoke, mold spores or animal dander, air-conditioners are often less effective by comparison. Misleading and confusing claims in this regard are common. An air-conditioner may contain a mechanical or impingement filter, but the size of the particle which this removes depends upon the size of the openings in the filter. Larger dust particles and pollens may be removed by high-quality, fibrous filters; smaller allergenic particles may not. Before you purchase a unit, if you desire air purification as well as cooling, ascertain whether 95 per cent of pollen particles in the 10- to 20-micron range are removed. Ideally, filters should remove particles that are one micron in size or less. If smoke can be seen to pass through the machine, it is possibly not suitable for allergic persons.

## What do air-conditioners do?

They cool the air and dehumidify the atmosphere in a room or home. They make a room more comfortable, especially if the windows and doors are kept closed as is recommended when using a separate unit to purify the air. Some will remove pollens and various other air particles depending upon the quality of the filter and the size of the particle. Better-quality room models have a switch indicating either *ventilate* or *fresh air*, which allows about 10 to 15 per cent outside air to enter the room. These same machines would also usually have a switch indicating *recirculate*, which means that no fresh air is brought into the room. Another switch is sometimes marked *exhaust*, which means that cooled air can be forced from the room.

Air-conditioners often become contaminated with molds, especially after not being used all winter. If a moldy smell is noticed when the machine is first started, clean all removable parts with aqueous Zephiran chloride.

## Which type of air-conditioner is best?

If you purchase a room air-conditioner, try to obtain one which will recirculate and cool the air within the room, rather than the type which will continually circulate outside air (and pollen). If the machine has a switch indicating *recirculate* versus *ventilate* or *fresh air*, it should be kept on *recirculate*.

Central air-conditioners circulate and cool inside air and, combined with a central electrostatic-precipitation air-purifying unit, these machines would therefore continually remove pollen, some air contamination, excessive moisture and heat. The plastic, motor oils or oil or gas energy in these units can cause symptoms in most chemically sensitive persons.

## If finances are a problem, how can you inexpensively make your child's bedroom air clean and comfortable?

The best method would be to place your allergic child (or children) in a small bedroom, use a small, portable, electronic air purifier and install a large fan to circulate the air.

If a small air-conditioner is not too much of an expense, buy the type which can circulate and cool only the air in the bedroom.

It is not sensible for parents, in their great desire to help their child, to immediately install a furnace air-conditioner, electronic air-filter and humidifier. This can easily cost thousands, and can make some children worse.

### Are air-depollution units, air-cleaners and air-conditioners tax deductible?

Usually, but not necessarily. Your physician can give you a statement that these items were recommended solely for medical purposes if, in his opinion, they were essential for your child's health. The final decision, however, rests with the Internal Revenue Service.

## HOBBIES

### Which hobbies can cause allergies?

This list could be as long as a list of hobbies. Some major ones which could cause allergic symptoms are:

    Growing plants involving soil possibly contaminated with molds

    Sewing or knitting making use of wool, angora, mohair or synthetic fabrics which could cause difficulty

    Printing using flaxseed in the printer's ink

    Raising any pets with fur or feathers

    Playing wind instruments that have a reed mouthpiece which can cause symptoms, either because of the reed or shellac on the reed

    Playing stringed instruments requiring rosin on the bow

    Working with wood or some types of paints or similar substances

    Use of hay or straw for decoration or crafts

    Gourmet cooking using dried herbs or roots.

(Any odor can cause some patients to become ill.)

### Can glue cause allergies?

It certainly can, especially if it is made from fish. Such glues are usually tan or brownish in color. Contact with products which could be glued together, such as boxes, books, toys (model planes) or even "old" furniture, can possibly cause difficulty. The glue dust can contain enough fish ingredients to cause symptoms. Children with this problem can usually use a white paste without difficulty. The clear, colorless glues or cements used for model airplanes can cause symptoms because of their odor (see Appendix, p. 266). Licking stamps and envelopes can cause symptoms in corn-sensitive patients.

## CHEMICAL SENSITIVITIES

**How can you suspect which patient has a chemical sensitivity?**
One clue is that affected persons often have a keen sense of smell and a profound dislike of specific odors. However, just as with some food-sensitive patients, the chemically-sensitive may sometimes crave the odor to which they are sensitive. The person who likes the smell of a new car, fresh paint or glue may be giving a clue that odors are a problem, and avoidance of chemical exposure might be advisable before obviously health-related symptoms arise.

**Does everyone need to have a chemically-free home?**
Fortunately, no. Many patients who have allergies appear to respond favorably if their bedrooms, in particular, are made relatively allergy-free. To make a home chemically-free is an awesome and expensive task. Such patients usually have their problem diagnosed in special, chemically-free hospital units and are often restored to tolerable health in about six days. They remain well until challenged by specific chemicals or foods in the controlled hospital unit. Once these patients return home, however, their problems return unless they are able to live in a chemically-free home.

## TESTS FOR CHEMICAL SENSITIVITIES

Test the following only if you or a family member are *normally* exposed to the listed items at home, school or work. Select a time when symptoms are minimal. Never test yourself. Someone must time the test and observe for possible reactions. Do the test in a room which can be avoided for several hours if a reaction occurs. Discuss the test with your physician first. Test only if he approves.

Schedule the test so that it is midway between meals, at 11:00 A.M. or 3:00 P.M. Do no more than one test per day. Observe for any change in activity, behavior, or the onset of symptoms, for example, flushing, pallor, stuffiness, headache, muscle ache, dizziness, and so on. Check the pulse before the test. If any test produces symptoms, stop exposure immediately. Breathe fresh air or oxygen. Take one teaspoon of baking soda in two glasses of water. If no reaction is noticed after the specified time of exposure, stop the test. Continue to watch the patient for an additional half hour for delayed reactions. Take the pulse for one full minute every ten minutes during the entire test. A pulse increase of 12 to 20 may indicate a sensitivity to the item tested. Ask a nurse to show you how to check a pulse, if you are unsure.

Shellac, turpentine, creosol, kerosene, gasoline, acetone (nail polish remover), perfume (test each one separately), underarm deodorant, hair, body, bathroom or kitchen aerosols, phenol (Lysol), floor wax, furniture or shoe polish, camphor, pesticide, herbicide, insecticide, liquid paint or glue:

Test each item individually.
Place a few drops or small spray on a blotter.
Expose patient for 20 minutes at 2 feet.

Clorox, ammonia, scouring powder:
Test one at a time.
Place one tablespoon in one cup water.
Expose patient for 20 minutes at 4 feet.

Foam rubber, polyurethane, soft plastic or plastic polyethylene food or garment bags, freshly cleaned or new polyester clothing:
Test each item individually.
Expose patient for approximately 20 minutes at 2 feet.

Gas fumes:
Sit 2 to 3 feet from a stove which has lighted gas burners and lighted oven for 20 to 30 minutes.
Have doors to room closed.

Tobacco:
Sit in a room filled with tobacco smoke without eating or drinking for 20 minutes.

Newsprint or chemically treated paper (mimeograph, copying machine):
Keep freshly printed paper 6 inches from face for approximately 20 minutes.

Soap, detergent, or fabric softener:

Soak washcloth in usual concentration for each item. Squeeze out excess fluid.
Keep item 6 inches from face for 20 minutes.
Test each item separately.

Exhaust fumes:
Stand near busy bus stop for 15 to 20 minutes.

Electric blanket or heating pad fumes:

Place either on chest for 20 minutes.

As plastic-coated wires heat, odors are emitted.

Motor oils:

Stand near small motor for ten minutes.

Mothballs or crystals:

Expose patient at 6 feet for 20 minutes.

Carpet, linoleum, tile, upholstered furniture, mattresses or bed sheets:

Sit directly upon item for 20 to 30 minutes. Does portion of body in contact with item tingle or feel different?

Food Coloring:

Do not test for dyes without a physician's supervision. Severe reactions have been noted in some adults. Do not test for dyes unless all colored foods, beverages and medicine are normally taken without obvious symptoms. Place one drop of red, grocery store food coloring under the tongue. Hold it for one minute. Then swallow. Test other colors (yellow, blue), one each day. Observe for 20 minutes. If the above is negative, give one tablespoon of colored Jell-O or artificially colored beverage at five-day intervals. Observe for 20 minutes after ingestion.

Tests for chemical sensitivities courtesy of Natalie Golos and Francis Golos Golbitz *Coping With Your Allergies*, Simon and Schuster, N.Y.: 1979.

# CHAPTER 9

# Food allergies beyond infancy

WARNING! Never feed your child any food which caused a violent reaction when eaten previously.

## SYMPTOMS CAUSED BY FOODS

**Which symptoms can be caused by food allergies?**

Any allergic symptom can. Usually foods cause eczema, asthma, nose, eye and ear allergies (secretory otitis), hives or body swellings and digestive problems. The latter could be manifested as excess mucus, excess gas (rectal or oral), halitosis, abdominal pain, bloating, loose bowel movements, constipation or nausea. Food allergies also can cause mouth ulcers, irritability, fluid weight gain, styes, headaches, cold sores, a geographic tongue (mottled, irregular, denuded areas on tongue), anal or rectal itching, aching joints or muscles, inattentiveness, fatigue or behavior problems. Shock or fainting, numb extremities, bed wetting, tingling and restless legs can be due to food problems.

Allergy is not the only cause of a digestive upset, so this should be considered only *after* your physician has investigated other frequent causes of intestinal problems. One of the most common is abdominal pain or discomfort related to constipation. This type of pain disappears shortly after the bowels are moved. Surgical problems also can cause digestive difficulties.

**Is it possible for one food to cause one symptom and another to cause a different symptom?**

Yes. For example, milk may be the cause of asthma, but a child's eczema may clear only when chocolate is eliminated. The same food, wheat cereal, for example, may cause eczema during infancy, asthma at three years, hyperactivity and behavior problems at six, and headaches, muscle aches, bellyaches and fatigue at twenty. In this case the shock organ has changed from the skin to the chest, brain and body, but the same food is responsible for all the symptoms.

### When testing to see if a food causes allergy, what symptom do you look for?

It depends upon the individual child. Be alert for the disappearance of any symptom when a certain food is not being eaten and for the reappearance of this symptom when the food is again included in your child's diet. The manifestation of allergy could be as pronounced as hay fever or asthma, or as subtle as a change in disposition, abdominal discomfort or a headache. Symptoms may occur in 15 minutes or several hours later and may last for hours, or two or three days.

### What are examples of extreme food allergy?

This type of allergy may occur from the mere odor of certain foods called osmyls, or from contact with minute amounts of food. Some children are so allergic to eggs that if a mother were to crack an egg in the kitchen while her youngster was in another room, the child might immediately have symptoms of allergy. Such an extreme allergy is also apparent in some children upon exposure to the smell of nuts, fish or buckwheat. Some children begin to wheeze merely when passing a nut counter in a store, or because of an odor of fish in a market or cafeteria. If a child is exceptionally allergic to peanut butter, other children in the family should not eat it. Just opening the jar could cause illness. It has been said that a child who is very allergic to eggs cannot, for example, kiss someone who has just eaten eggs because the minute amount of egg lingering on the lips or breath could cause a reaction. This degree of sensitivity is, fortunately, rare. Any child who is extremely allergic to a food should wear a name tag stating that this type of food causes difficulty.

Although it is unusual, some children who are very highly sensitive to eggs cannot use an egg shampoo because this contact can cause itching of the scalp or possibly other allergic symptoms. Certain food-type cosmetics, *e.g.,* cucumber in face cream, can cause similar problems.

## SPECIFIC FOODS WHICH CAUSE ALLERGIES

### How often is a food the cause of a child's allergies?

Food allergy seems to be a frequent cause of children's allergies, although many allergists believe that only five per cent of allergic children are sensitive to a specific food. This type of allergy is difficult to recognize and diagnose. Food can be the sole cause of an allergic problem in infants. Foods appear to cause many symptoms in children or adults which are misdiagnosed as psychological problems.

### How many foods can cause a child's allergy?

They can vary from one to several. If a child has many foods which truly provoke allergic symptoms, a physician's help is needed. If this is not possible, a Rotary Diet might give the answers.

### At what age does a food allergy first occur?

At any age. Most food allergies are noted in the first year of life and may disappear within a year or two, although some may persist indefinitely. Older persons can develop allergies at any time, but occasionally these also disappear after several months or years for no apparent reason. Very strong allergies to foods, however, such as those to eggs, fish or nuts, tend to last for many years or for life.

### Can any food cause allergy?

Yes, but some foods are more apt to cause this problem than others. (See p. 272.)

### Which foods are most apt to cause allergies after infancy?

Milk, wheat, eggs, fish, nuts, chocolate, cola, sugar, coffee, pork products, tomato, food dyes, peas, peanuts, citrus products, celery, mustard, corn (popcorn), fresh berries, cantaloupe, and spices such as cinnamon and nutmeg. Fresh foods can cause symptoms if they are contaminated with insecticides or chemicals. If you can eat a food such as an apple that is organically grown, but not when it is sold in the usual store, your problem is due to chemical contamination of food. Canned, frozen or pre-packaged foods may contain preservatives, dyes and additives which can cause symptoms in some people. Flour may cause symptoms only when it is sifted and breathed into the lungs, but these persons can often ingest wheat products without difficulty.

### Which foods are least apt to cause allergy?

Lamb, rice, barley, pears, peaches, lettuce, carrots, squash, sweet potatoes, oats, grapes and poi. In some patients, however, any of these foods can cause symptoms. An infant is often changed from wheat to rice cereal to eliminate some allergic problem. If he improves, rice is continued in the diet. Occasionally, rice may later cause allergies and is never suspected because it previously helped the child to improve and because it seldom causes allergies. Finally, when rice is eliminated, the desired improvement is noted.

*No* food is to be considered entirely safe, and an allergist who is knowledgeable about food allergy is the best person to evaluate the more difficult problems.

### Which kinds of fish cause allergies?

Any type. Persons allergic to mackerel supposedly cannot eat tuna. Those sensitive to salmon cannot eat trout. Other persons cannot eat other varieties, such as whitefish, cod, halibut, haddock, sole, pike, perch, etc. Lobster, crab and shrimp are crustaceans and an allergy to one often indicates an allergy to all, even though the others may never have been eaten. Oysters, scallops and clams belong to the mollusk family and, again, a child or adult could be allergic to any or all of these.

### What clue sometimes signifies fish or egg allergy?

Some children have allergies only on Friday night or Saturday morning. This is frequently due to eating fish or eggs on Fridays or when observing religious holidays. Some children who do not actually consume fish become ill each weekend because of the smell of fish which other family members have cooked or brought into the house.

### Which food additives cause allergy?

Almost anything added to a food can cause symptoms: Anti-oxidants, buffers, color additives, emulsifiers, flavorings, minerals, neutralizing substances, preservatives, pesticides, stabilizers, sweetening agents (artificial or other), thickeners (pectin, tragacanth or acacia) or vitamins. One of these items could account for the reason that a food processed by one manufacturer might cause allergic symptoms while the same food prepared by another does not. A reaction to one of these is most difficult to detect and would probably require the aid of an allergist. Medicines often contain similar additives. Newer, controversial methods of skin testing claim that sensitivities to these items can be diagnosed.

### Can molds on foods cause allergies?

Certain foods that are grown in damp places (mushrooms), aged (steaks) or preserved (smoked or pickled products) can cause symptoms in some children. Melons could have molds on the outside. Certain cheeses could have molds in them causing difficulty. Dried or candied fruits (apricots, raisins, prunes) also could be similarly contaminated.

## How can a vitamin allergy be determined?

If your child's reaction to a vitamin is not extreme, it should be quite simple to determine the cause. Check the composition of the vitamin which seems to create an allergic symptom. If its composition is complex, buy a few samples of simpler vitamin mixtures that contain only three or four vitamins. See if these also precipitate allergies. When you have narrowed down the vitamin preparation to one which contains only a few ingredients, buy a few individual vitamin types from the druggist and test each. For example, if the vitamin mixture tablet or liquid causing difficulty contained vitamin A, $B_1$, $B_2$ and C, obtain a few of each of these. By giving each type singly for three days, you should be able to determine which is the problem component. Vitamin $B_1$ is also called thiamine hydrochloride, $B_2$ is riboflavin and C is ascorbic acid. If individual vitamin ingredients (such as A, $B_1$, $B_2$, or C) do not cause an allergic symptom while a vitamin mixture containing these does, ask your physician's help in determining whether the dye, flavor or sweeteners used in this vitamin tablet could be the source of difficulty. Vitamins are available that are free of corn, sugar and food coloring. (See Appendix IV.)

## Which vitamins cause allergy?

Cod liver oil capsules cannot be taken by children allergic to fish; vitamin B sometimes has been implicated as a rare cause of allergy. Water-soluble vitamins A, C, and D seldom cause allergy. Dyes, sugar, corn and artificial flavors can cause symptoms in some patients. (See pp. 287–288 for list of where to buy allergy-free vitamins.)

## Can yeast cause allergy?

Some children cannot eat baked foods which are made with a yeast dough. Fermented drinks such as wine or beer could cause difficulty. Pickled foods could also be a factor. Yeast in vitamins can cause allergy, especially in mold-sensitive patients.

## What special circumstances can make a child develop a food allergy?

Feeding a child highly allergenic foods (see Appendix, p. 272) during an episode of diarrhea or for a few days afterward can make him more prone to develop an allergy to the foods recently eaten. Diarrhea makes the intestines more porous or open, and food absorption can be greater at this time. If foods are not thoroughly digested, large allergenic proteins are absorbed, instead of small, altered, protein-like particles which are less likely to cause allergic sensitivity.

If solid foods are added to a newborn's diet too early in infancy, the immature intestines are more apt to allow undigested foods to pass into the blood. This would increase the chance of developing food allergies.

A large excess of a food or eating a food more often than every four days also can make someone more prone to develop a new food allergy.

## SKIN TESTS FOR FOODS

### How reliable are skin tests for food?

*Traditional* food skin tests are very unreliable. A few foods such as fish or nuts might show correlation between a decidedly positive skin test and an actual allergy when the food is eaten. For most foods, however, the correlation or relationship is very inconclusive. One reason for this is that the allergist cannot test for digested and cooked foods. It is mainly the protein portion of a food which causes allergy, and cooking or digestion changes this protein to such a degree that a skin test (for example, of a raw egg white) on the arm or back simply is not accurate. Eggs are most often eaten in a cooked, rather than raw, form. *Newer,* controversial methods to skin-test and treat food allergy are presently available. I find them accurate and helpful. (See Appendix V.)

### Why do allergists perform *traditional* skin tests for food if they are so unreliable?

At times they might give some indication of a food which is related to allergic symptoms. Skin tests may help to guide the physician in selecting possible allergic foods for dietary testing. If only one or two foods cause large skin test reactions, these can be checked by omitting them for a week to see if the allergic symptoms improve and then restoring them to the diet to see if allergies recur. *If all or most of the food skin tests are positive,* it could indicate multiple food allergies. (See Appendix VI.) There is slight evidence to show that scratch skin tests for raw foods may be more accurate than intradermal or needle skin tests, but in general most skin tests for foods are unreliable unless the newer methods are used. Several skin tests must be done using 1:5 dilutions of a single food extract before a diagnosis can be made.

### Can allergy-injection treatments be successfully given for food allergies?

This form of therapy is felt by many allergists to be ineffective. There are, however, a growing number of allergists who claim success using the provocation and neutralization injection method for treating food allergy. I was very skeptical but now find that the newer methods are effective in enabling patients to eat, in moderation, foods which previously caused allergic symptoms.

## VARIABLES AFFECTING FOOD ALLERGIES

**How soon after a food is eaten can symptoms be expected to occur?**

This would vary greatly depending upon the degree of sensitivity. If the allergy is extreme, a reaction occurs in seconds. Other foods might not cause symptoms for several days after being eaten. Some foods cause symptoms several hours later. A food may have to be digested and a certain blood level of this digested food attained before symptoms are evident.

Some foods gradually accumulate in the body and after the food is eaten for a week or so allergic symptoms are noted. This can occur with milk, wheat or eggs. Symptoms do not occur suddenly after re-adding such foods, but possibly a month or so later you may notice your child wheezing more often than before restoration of the suspected foods. Symptoms reappear so gradually that the food is not suspected as the cause.

Fish, berries, nuts and uncooked or partially cooked eggs often cause immediate allergic reactions. Milk, cooked eggs, beef, white potato, orange, chocolate, wheat, corn, pork, peas and peanuts are somewhat more apt to cause delayed reactions, noted several hours after these foods are eaten. Exceptions, however, would not be unusual. In any child who is allergic to a food, the interval between eating different foods and the appearance of the symptoms may not be constant. One child may have asthma ten minutes after eating fish and hay fever two hours after eating pizza. Another child can have asthma ten hours after eating fish and hay fever two minutes after eating pizza. The time interval between eating the food and noting a particular symptom, however, can vary with fatigue, stress, emotion, the way the food was prepared, hormones, and the frequency of ingestion and the amount eaten at one time.

**May a child crave a food which is causing his allergy?**

Yes. Often the offending food is a favorite, such as milk, chocolate or peanut butter. In other children, however, there is a natural aversion to any form of contact with a food to which they are allergic. Again, milk, chocolate and orange juice are common examples. Adults with food sensitivity often crave coffee, wheat, cola, chocolate or beer.

**If a child refuses to eat a certain food, does it mean the child is allergic to it?**

No. Children with allergies can have food likes and dislikes just as any other child. In the case of an allergic child, however, no attempt should be made to force the child to eat some food which he does not want to eat. It is possible for a child to be extremely allergic to a food which could cause a severe allergic reaction if only a little of it were eaten or smelled. The problem is to decide whether a child is asserting his individuality by refusing a particular food or if he is in some way able to sense his allergy to the food which causes him to avoid it. There is no safe immediate solution to this problem.

Some children refuse to eat chocolate or ice cream. This is unusual and could point to an allergy. On the other hand, children, like adults, have natural food preferences and a child's refusal to eat squash or liver, for instance, would not be significant of an allergic tendency.

**Can the quantity or quality of a single food which is eaten be a factor related to an allergy?**

Yes. A child very allergic to milk, for example, might not be able to drink even a few drops; another might be able to drink one glass a day, and still another might be able to drink three glasses a day before allergic symptoms appear.

Quality refers to the form in which a food is eaten. In general, cooked foods cause less difficulty than uncooked foods. A child might be able to tolerate a small amount of egg in cake or cookies. Another might be able to eat half a hard-boiled egg. Some children can eat one scrambled egg each day but might become ill from more than one. Eggnogs or an egg white frosting cannot be eaten by a child who cannot tolerate uncooked egg protein.

**Is it possible to have a food allergy which would cause symptoms only at certain seasons?**

This is indeed possible. Some allergenic substances can be tolerated in tiny amounts without causing symptoms. If, however, the threshold for a child's symptoms is exceeded, the allergic problem becomes evident. Certain foods plus dust in the winter can cause a stuffy nose, while foods alone in the summer may not. Children are exposed to much less house dust in the summer months. There are some patients who cannot eat melon or even bananas during the ragweed season. At other times these foods are no problem. (See p. 15.) There is also evidence that hay fever patients with an itchy throat from bananas or melon during the ragweed season are more prone to pollen asthma than others.

**If a child is allergic to a food, must that food never be eaten?**

Of course not. Your common sense will tell you what to do. The treatment should never be worse than the disease. If a child has a few hives from chocolate and wants a chocolate cake for his birthday, it is certainly all right. Give the child an antihistamine and Alka-Seltzer, *in gold foil,* and don't worry. However, if chocolate causes severe asthma and your child needs to be hospitalized, or is up all night after one small piece of cake or candy, it certainly should be avoided.

**If a food causes a *serious* problem, should your child purposely be fed or skin-tested with this food?**

No. If you are absolutely sure about it, why cause your child to be ill? The food which seems to be causing a serious problem should be avoided *in all forms.*

**Can similar foods cause allergy?**

Yes. At times patients are allergic to one certain food, but closely related foods also can cause difficulty. For example, oranges might cause severe nasal allergies while lemons might cause only mild hay fever. Both of these foods are citrus fruits. Foods can be classified in certain families and a child who is allergic to peanuts, for example, may possibly have difficulty when eating peas, or any type of beans, or licorice, because all of these are legumes. If any similar foods are found to cause symptoms, these should also be avoided.

In regard to the pea family, it should also be mentioned that honey is often gathered from plants in this family and some children who cannot eat foods such as peas or peanuts cannot eat honey for this reason. (See Appendix II giving this information and the names of related foods.)

**What can be done if a child accidentally eats a food to which he is very allergic?**

Often a child will vomit immediately after a slight taste of the offending food and this is nature's way of helping him. If the food is truly dangerous and your child has not vomited, you can put your finger down his throat to precipitate vomiting. Be sure your child does not aspirate or swallow any material when he vomits. Small children can be turned upside down so that they will not choke on the vomited material. If your child can't vomit, or has vomited, immediately give both an asthma medicine and an antihistamine if these are available; also give Alka-Seltzer, *in gold foil,* or baking soda. Rush your child to the nearest physician or hospital, *after* doing the above, if there is the slightest reason for concern.

### Can eating a food to which a child is extremely allergic cause death?

Yes. A danger sign would be swelling of the back of the tongue or throat. If this begins to happen, the child usually becomes hoarse. If you have an antihistamine or asthma medicine, immediately give your child both, and Alka-Seltzer, *in gold foil,* in the proper dosage, and rush him to the nearest hospital. Such extreme food allergy is, fortunately, very rare but could occur after such foods as eggs, nuts, fish or buckwheat are eaten.

### If a food is causing significant symptoms, how long should it be avoided?

The food should not be eaten for at least two months and in some patients for six months or longer. It can be re-added to the diet at intervals of two to about six months to determine if the food can be eaten without causing undesirable reactions. Responses to foods often change in time. Eat the problem food at five-day intervals.

If a food caused a severe, alarming reaction, it should *not* be tested or eaten again. If at some future time this particular food is *accidentally* eaten without difficulty, then it *probably* can be consumed and will not cause symptoms. It is possible, however, for a certain brand of a food to cause a severe reaction while another brand does not. The cause could be due to a food additive or to a difference in the method of processing. Be certain to check with your doctor before re-adding foods of this type. Allergies to eggs, nuts, buckwheat, and particularly fish, may last a lifetime.

### If a child has one food allergy, is he apt to have others?

Yes. If a child seems better when one food is eliminated from his diet, but if the allergic symptoms do not stop completely, there could be more foods complicating the problem.

### If a food causes digestive problems, is it always because of allergies?

No. It could be due to a pharmacological effect such as bowel problems with prunes or baked beans. Some persons or families cannot tolerate greasy foods. Others lack specific enzymes necessary to digest certain foods such as grains or milk products. Certain milk sugars can cause almost constant diarrhea in some infants (and adults) on this basis. Foods can also be contaminated with bacteria or spoiled and this could cause symptoms when eaten and would be completely unrelated to allergy. Improperly home-canned products could cause illness from

toxic substances. If your child always has frothy, greasy, foul-smelling
bowel movements, he may have fibrocystic disease which is unrelated
to a food allergy.

In infants, allergy is sometimes said to be the cause of a baby's
digestive problems when other entirely unrelated factors are actually at
fault. The baby may not tolerate a formula because it was too hot or
cold, made incorrectly, because the holes in the nipple were too large
or too small, because he was fed too quickly or positioned improperly,
or because he was not burped often enough or adequately. Your pediatrician can help solve these problems.

## WHEN AND HOW SHOULD PARENTS CHECK
## FOR FOOD ALLERGIES?

**Is there any truly reliable method of checking for a food allergy?**

Many have been attempted. A clinical dietary trial seems to be the
most accurate. Remove a food and see if symptoms disappear. Restore
the food and observe if symptoms recur. It is also presently possible
to detect with a blood examination (RAST test) extreme food sensitivities which occur *immediately* after contact with certain foods. We have
no blood test, however, for certain types of immediate and most delayed
food reactions. There is also a new skin test for foods—the Bioassay
Titration Method. One often can provoke the exact allergic symptoms
which a food causes with one dilution, and promptly eliminate these
symptoms with another dilution, of the same food. These newer methods are not widely used, accepted or available as yet, but preliminary
evidence of their effectiveness is most encouraging.

**Do you need a physician's help to attempt dietary studies?**

Not necessarily.

If a symptom caused by a food is not life-threatening, an attempt can
be made to test single foods without any danger. No experiment should
be made without the aid of an allergist to check a food which could be
causing a serious allergic reaction. If you are trying to eliminate several
foods or many foods for more than one or two weeks, a physician
should be consulted so that your child's proper growth is assured.

**How difficult are dietary trials?**

You can do dietary studies if you are determined to help your child,
but determination you will need. You must understand *all* the possible
sources of the food which is to be eliminated from the diet. If, for

example, a child is allergic to milk and is being given pudding or most breads, the child is actually receiving milk and is on no diet at all. A mother must read all labels on *every* food her child eats. The family must be patient and realize that the physician is not being petty but attempting to make a child well. Siblings must realize that they are not doing the allergic child a favor to sneak him the "forbidden food," since this will only make impossible or greatly delay determination of the cause of the allergy. The whole family must understand that, at times, a speck of the offending food can possibly cause symptoms.

### When should dietary trials be attempted?

Make the studies when a child's allergic symptoms seem to be stable and minimal. If a child's breathing is nasal and he needs an antihistamine twice a day, this is the child's "normal baseline." It would indicate a food allergy if: (1) when the food is omitted, antihistamines could be discontinued and, (2) when the food was re-added and eaten in excess at a five-day interval, the need for antihistamines markedly increased.

The food in question must be omitted from the diet and *re-added* to determine if the observed result was from food or, for example, from a coincidental infection.

Easter time is excellent for checking a child for chocolate allergy. Omit chocolate for five to 12 days before Easter and give the usual amount on the holiday. If the symptoms are negligible until chocolate is eaten, but then flare up, this would be highly suggestive of an allergy to cocoa (or sugar or corn) in chocolate candy.

### When should dietary trials *not* be attempted?

1. Avoid these trials if your child has an infection. Infections often make allergies worse and if you are checking to see if a food causes allergic symptoms, you cannot interpret the effect. Dietary studies should also be avoided when an infection seems to be passing throughout your family.

2. During pollen seasons, it is often difficult to deduce whether foods or pollens cause a flare-up of symptoms.

3. If your child has had recent surgery or severe trauma, food studies should be delayed.

4. Attempt dietary studies after your child's room and your home have been made as allergy-free as possible. You may find that this alone will solve your child's problem. Dietary studies would be indicated first only if your child's year-round symptoms persist in spite of your making your home allergy-free.

5. If your child is thin and undernourished, do not attempt to do *any* dietary manipulation without a physician's help.

6. If your child is violently allergic to a food, attempt no study of the food without your allergist's advice. This is particularly true for egg, milk, buckwheat, nut or fish allergies.

7. Avoid testing if you will be traveling or eating in restaurants.

8. Try not to test for food allergies near birthdays, holidays or special occasions.

**Why is a single-food dietary study often unrewarding?**

Suppose a child is allergic to milk, egg and wheat. If milk is omitted from the diet, the wheat and eggs would continue to cause allergic symptoms. When milk is re-added, the wheat and eggs could still be partly responsible for allergic symptoms. This situation makes it difficult to interpret the importance of milk. For this reason, if a child is thought to have several food allergies, it is best to place the child on a diet of a few foods which seldom cause allergy. Single foods can be re-added after improvement is observed. Offending foods are more easily determined in this manner.


# HOW TO CARRY OUT DIETARY TRIALS


**What are the three most practical diets to detect food allergies?**

1. A *Simple Elimination Diet:* helpful for a *single* food problem.

2. A *Multiple Elimination Diet:* helpful for an allergy to *several* common foods.

3. A *Rotary Diet:* helpful for infants or adults who are sensitive to *innumerable* foods.

**How is the *Simple Elimination Diet* carried out?**

Merely stop eating the suspect food in *every* form for a maximum of 12 days. (Diet lists for common individual foods are listed on pp. 269 to 271.) After 12 days (or sooner, if the symptoms disappear) eat the food which has been avoided. If a true food sensitivity exists, symptoms should recur within about one hour after eating a normal-sized portion on an empty stomach. On occasion, an offending food has to be eaten for two or three days before symptoms recur. It is sometimes possible to relieve food symptoms within 20 minutes by taking Alka-Seltzer Antacid Formula, without aspirin (*gold foil*), shortly after symptoms are noted.

**Which *Multiple Elimination Diet* might help detect allergies to several common major foods?**

The proposed diet is in two distinct parts. Have your physician's permission before you try this diet.

# PART 1

**How do you use the first part of the diet?**

During the first week, the following foods are omitted in *all* forms. Milk and dairy products, wheat (bread, cake, cookies, baked goods), eggs, corn, sugar, chocolate (cocoa or cola), peas (peanut butter), citrus (orange, lemon, lime, grapefruit), food coloring, food additives and preservatives. Most meats, fruits and vegetables can be eaten. No luncheon meats, sausage, ham, bacon, peas or corn are allowed. (The "allowed" foods are listed on pages 156 and 157.) If there is some question about a specific food, do not eat it. Keep detailed records in the diaries found on pages 148 to 149 of exactly what is eaten. If you or your child are better in a week or less, immediately begin Part 2 of the diet. If you are not better within a week, try continuing Part 1 of the diet for a second week. Occasionally, a patient does not show improvement for about fourteen days.

If Part 1 of the diet has not helped by the fourteenth day, this particular diet is probably not the answer for your child (or you). Re-check the diet records for the initial week of the diet. Were *only* the allowed foods eaten?

Occasionally, a person is worse during Part 1 of the diet. If this happens, immediately stop the diet. A frequent cause is that the patient has begun to eat an excessive amount of an unsuspected offending food. For example, a child who substitutes grape juice for milk may find he is much worse, if grape juice is the cause of his symptoms.

Most patients who are going to respond favorably to the diet do so about the sixth or seventh day. Some may begin to improve as early as the second, or as late as the fourteenth day.

## RECORDS FOR
### Part 1
### *MULTIPLE ELIMINATION DIET—FOOD DIARY*

Record EVERYTHING eaten (gum, medications, etc.) each day.
Record in RED when any symptom begins each day.

|                | Day 1 | Day 2 | Day 3 | Day 4 | Day 5 | Day 6 | Day 7 |
|----------------|-------|-------|-------|-------|-------|-------|-------|
| **BREAKFAST**  |       |       |       |       |       |       |       |
| **SNACKS**     |       |       |       |       |       |       |       |
| **LUNCH**      |       |       |       |       |       |       |       |

SNACKS

DINNER

SNACKS

COMMENT

Used by permission of Syntex Laboratories. From the booklet *Food Sensitivity Diets.*
© 1978 by Doris J. Rapp.

**Special tips for the *Multiple Elimination Diet*.**

The "allowed" foods can be selected, combined and eaten in any quantity.

For a beverage, you can mix the allowed fruits in the blender with spring water and honey or pure maple syrup.

Your child's usual medications can be taken during the diet. If your child improves, you may find the medicine is needed less often by the end of the first week. Try to use only white pills (crushed for small children and placed in apple sauce or mashed potatoes) or colorless liquids. Most liquid medications contain corn, sugar and dyes which can cause symptoms in some children. Check with your physician about any questions you may have.

Once you determine which foods cause specific symptoms, you must discuss the problem with your physician. Some foods cannot be omitted for indefinite periods of time if a child's nutrition is to be maintained.

Do not try the diet when your child has an infection or is receiving an antibiotic.

Although the symptoms may vary, food sensitivities are often evident in several family members. One child might have headaches, another a stuffy nose, and a third, hyperactivity. The same food, *e.g.*, milk, may be a problem for several generations of a family. For this reason, make cooking easier by placing the entire family on the diet. A fringe benefit may be that you may relieve some "emotional or learn-to-live-with" health problems caused by a certain food in several family members.

If your child has asthma, add the test food back into the diet with extreme care. It is possible that an unsuspected food could precipitate a sudden severe asthma attack. Have asthma medications on hand during Part 2 of the diet.

If your child refuses the diet, try offering a reward. Promise a gala party if there is no cheating and if it is obvious that the child is truly trying very hard to cooperate in every way. The party should take place after both parts of the diet are completed. Give your child the foods which caused symptoms and this will be a double check confirming the effect of these foods on your child.

# PART 2

## How do you use the second part of the diet?

During Part 2 of the diet, one food is eaten in excess each day as suggested on pages 154 and 155. Keep detailed records of each day on page 152. Start with a teaspoon or ½ cup of the test food item and double the amount eaten every few hours, so that by the end of the day more than the normal amount has been ingested. Do any symptoms suddenly reappear? If there are no undesirable symptoms during the day, during the night or the next morning before breakfast, the food tested the day before is probably all right and may be eaten whenever desired. If the test food causes symptoms, stop eating it in all forms until you can secure the advice of your physician. Do not add another test food until the symptoms from the previous food test have subsided. Usually a parent will notice that symptoms are caused by a food within a few hours, and if Alka-Seltzer Antacid Formula without aspirin (gold foil) or the usual allergy medications are taken, the symptoms will subside before the next test food is due to be added to the diet.

REMEMBER: If one of the listed foods causes a reaction (not helped by Alka-Seltzer in gold foil) which lasts for over 24 hours, DO NOT TRY another food until the reaction has entirely subsided.

Watch closely to see what happens each day. One food might cause a stuffy nose, the next no reaction at all, the next a bellyache. Some reactions occur immediately, others in several hours. If a food obviously causes symptoms, it should not be eaten. If you are uncertain whether a food causes symptoms, discontinue it until the other foods have been checked. Then give the patient the suspect food every five days and see if symptoms recur each time it is eaten.

# RECORDS FOR

## Part II

### MULTIPLE ELIMINATION DIET – FOOD DIARY

| | Day 8 | Day 9 | Day 10 | Day 11 | Day 12 | Day 13 | Day 14 | Day 15 | Day 16 | Day 17 |
|---|---|---|---|---|---|---|---|---|---|---|
| B R E A K F A S T | Excess milk, cottage cheese | Excess bread & wheat cereal (No preservatives) | Excess sugar (Sugar cubes) | Excess eggs | Excess cocoa | Excess dyed foods. Jell-O, fruited drinks, candy | Excess corn. Popcorn, whole kernel & corn flakes | Excess preservatives, baked goods, luncheon meats | Excess orange, grapefruit, lemon, lime | Excess peanut butter |
| S N A C K S | | | | | | | | | | |

| LUNCH | SNACKS | DINNER | COMMENT | |
|---|---|---|---|---|
| | | | | |

Used by permission of Syntex Laboratories. From the booklet *Food Sensitivity Diets*.

© 1978 by Doris J. Rapp.

## SPECIAL TIPS FOR PART 2 OF
### *MULTIPLE ELIMINATION DIET*

For Part 2 of diet—Tips to make adding food back into the patient's diet easier

| | |
|---|---|
| In Part 1 (days 1 to 7) you omitted foods. Now you add them back. | Below are suggestions to help you with each food. Don't add any food if you already know it causes a bad reaction. If in doubt, check with your doctor. |
| Milk—Day 8 | Give the patient lots of milk, cottage cheese and whipped cream sweetened with saccharin, sucaryl or honey. No butter, margarine or yellow cheese unless you are absolutely certain they contain NO yellow dyes. |
| Wheat—Day 9 | Add plain soda crackers or wheat cereal. If the patient had trouble from milk, be sure NOT to give milk products. Use Italian bread or kosher bread because these should not contain milk (casein or whey), but always read labels to be sure. You can bake if you like, but you must not use eggs or sugar. Remember, the patient can eat no dairy products or drink any milk if he seemed worse in any way on the milk day. If the milk caused no problem, milk products may be eaten. |
| Sugar—Day 10 | Give the patient sugar cubes to eat and add granulated sugar to the allowed foods. If milk or wheat caused trouble, they must be avoided or you can't tell if sugar is tolerated. |
| Egg—Day 11 | Add eggs in usual forms, cooked or as eggnog. Give custard. Remember, again, no wheat, milk or sugar can be consumed if any of these caused problems. |
| Cocoa—Day 12 | Add dark chocolate and cocoa. Only if the patient had no trouble with sugar and milk can you give milk chocolate. You can make hot chocolate with water, cocoa |

(pure Hershey's cocoa powder) and honey or an artificial sweetener. No candy bars are allowed because most contain corn. Remember, no milk, wheat, sugar, dyes or eggs are allowed if any of these caused symptoms.

| | |
|---|---|
| Food Coloring—Day 13 | Feed Jell-O, jelly or artifically colored fruit beverages (soda pop, Kool-Aid), Popsicles™ or cereal. Try to give lots of yellow, purple and red items because the patient might react to only one of these colors. Remember to avoid milk, wheat, Coca-Cola or sugar in all forms if any of these were a problem. If sugar caused symptoms, use honey, saccharin or sucaryl as a sweetener or buy dietetic pop and gelatin (D-Zerta). If milk, wheat or sugar were tolerated, they may be eaten. |
| Corn—Day 14 | Feed the patient corn, corn meal, corn flakes and popcorn. The latter can be made with salt and Crisco if food coloring was a problem. If milk, wheat, sugar, dyes, eggs or chocolate cause trouble, you can't give them on the same day you give corn. If you do, and the patient is worse, you won't be able to tell which is at fault. Do not use butter on popcorn if the patient has a milk sensitivity. |
| Preservatives—Day 15 | Read every label. Eat foods which contain any preservatives or food additives. In particular, eat luncheon meat, baloney, hot dogs, much bread or many baked goods and soups which contain preservatives and additives. |
| Citrus—Day 16 | Feed a large amount of lemon, lime, grapefruit or orange as fresh fruit, or in juice and gelatin. Avoid artificial dyes if food colors were a problem. Avoid gelatin if sugar was a problem. |
| Peanut Butter—Day 17 | Test for this only if it's a favorite food. Give lots of peanut butter or peanuts. Use Rykrisp if no wheat is allowed. Use *pure* peanut butter without additives. |

## MULTIPLE ELIMINATION DIET

| ALLOWED | FORBIDDEN |
|---|---|
| **CEREALS** Rice—Rice Puffs only Oats—Oatmeal made with honey Barley | **CEREALS** Foods containing wheat flour Corn Cereal mixtures (Granola) |
| **FRUITS** Any fresh fruit, except citrus Canned (if in their own juice and without artificial color, sugar or preservatives) | **FRUITS** Fresh frozen or canned** Citrus (orange, lemon, lime, grapefruit) |
| **BEVERAGES** Herb or other tea with honey, if desired Water Grape juice—bottled* (Welch's) Frozen apple juice* (Lincoln) Colorless diet cream soda Pure pineapple juice | **BEVERAGES** Milk or any type of dairy drink Fruit beverages except those so specified Kool-Aid Coffee Rich (yellow dye) 7 Up—Squirt—Teem Cola—Dr. Pepper |
| **SNACKS** Potato chips (no additives)—not canned Rykrisp crackers and pure honey Raisins (unsulfured) | **SNACKS** Corn chips—Fritos Chocolate or anything with cocoa Hard candy Ice cream or sherbert |

| ALLOWED | FORBIDDEN |
|---|---|
| **VEGETABLES** | **VEGETABLES** |
| Any *fresh* vegetables except corn and peas | Fresh frozen or canned** |
| French fries (homemade) | Corn |
| Potatoes | Mixed vegetables |
| | Peas |
| **MEATS** | **MEATS** |
| Chicken or turkey (non-basted) | Luncheon meats, wieners |
| Veal or beef | Bacon |
| Pork | Artificially colored hamburger or meat |
| Lamb | Ham |
| Fish, tuna | Dyed salmon, lobster |
| | Breaded meats |
| | Meats with stuffing |

\* Use only bottled which specifies no preservatives or additives.
\*\* If label specifies no food coloring or additives, these may be ingested.

| ALLOWED | FORBIDDEN |
|---|---|
| **MISCELLANEOUS** | **MISCELLANEOUS** |
| Pure honey | Sugar |
| Homemade vinegar and oil dressing | Bread, cake, cookies except on special recipes |
| Sea salt | Eggs |
| Pepper | Dyed (colored) vitamins, pills, mouth wash, toothpaste, medicines, cough syrups, etc. |
| Saccharin or artificial sweetener | Jelly or jam |
| Homemade soups | Jell-O |
| | Margarine or diet spreads (dyes and corn) |
| | Peanut butter— peanuts |
| | Sorbitol (corn) |

Used by permission of Syntex Laboratories. From the booklet *Food Sensitivity Diets*. © 1978 by Doris J. Rapp

**Special recipes for the** *Multiple Elimination Diet*

# Vegetables

### Oven-Browned Potatoes
Pare medium-sized potatoes and boil for 10 minutes. Place the parboiled potatoes around the roast in a roasting pan an hour or more before the meat is to be served. Turn the potatoes once or twice while they are roasting. If the potatoes do not brown sufficiently in the oven, they may be removed to a separate pan and placed under the broiler for a few minutes before serving. Browned potatoes may also be cooked in a separate pan with meat fat or melted Crisco or lard. Allow plenty of space between the potatoes so that they will brown, and roast at 375 degrees for about 1 hour.

### Candied Sweet Potatoes
| | |
|---|---|
| 4 | medium sweet potatoes |
| 1 | cup honey |
| 2 | tbs Crisco or lard |

Peel the potatoes and cut in half lengthwise. Arrange in a baking dish. Mix the remaining ingredients and pour over the potatoes. Bake at 375 degrees for 50 minutes.

### Spanish Rice
| | |
|---|---|
| ¼ | cup lard or Crisco |
| 1 | medium onion, thinly sliced |
| ½ | medium green pepper, diced |
| 1⅓ | cups Minute Rice |
| 1½ | cups hot water |
| 16 | oz homemade tomato sauce |
| 1 | tsp salt |
| | dash of pepper |

Melt fat in saucepan or skillet. Add onion, green pepper and rice. Cook and stir over high heat until slightly browned. Add remaining ingredients. Mix well. Bring quickly to a boil. Reduce heat and simmer, uncovered, for 5 minutes. Makes 4 servings.

# Salads

## Special Boiled Mayonnaise

| | |
|---|---|
| 1½ | tbs potato starch flour |
| ½ | tsp salt |
| ¼ | tsp dry mustard |
| 2 | tsp honey |
| ¼ | cup cold water |
| ¾ | cup boiling water |
| 1 | tbs white vinegar |
| ½ | cup vegetable oil (not corn) |
| | salt |
| | pepper |

Combine the potato starch, salt, dry mustard, and sugar in a saucepan and stir to a smooth paste with the ¼ cup of cold water. Add the boiling water and cook only until mixture is clear. Remove from heat and cool to lukewarm. Add the vinegar and oil, beating constantly. Season with salt and pepper. Makes 1¾ cups.

## Cole Slaw

| | |
|---|---|
| 1 | cup shredded cabbage |
| ½ | cup grated carrots |
| ¼ | cup minced green pepper |
| | special boiled mayonnaise |

Mix vegetables and blend with special boiled mayonnaise.

## Waldorf Salad

| | |
|---|---|
| 1 | apple, cored and chopped |
| | celery, chopped |
| 1 | tbs unsulfured raisins |
| | special boiled mayonnaise |

Combine apples, raisins, and celery. Mix lightly with special boiled mayonnaise until all pieces are coated. Chill.

# Salads (continued)

### French Dressing

| | |
|---|---|
| *1* | *cup vegetable oil* |
| ⅓ | *cup white vinegar* |
| *1* | *tsp salt* |
| *2* | *tsp honey* |
| *1* | *tsp paprika* |
| ⅛ | *tsp pepper* |
| *2* | *tsp water* |

In a jar combine all of the above ingredients. Cover tightly and shake well. Makes 1⅓ cups.

### Special Potato Salad

| | |
|---|---|
| | *sliced warm boiled potato* |
| | *fresh chopped chives (optional)* |
| | *chopped celery, fresh* |
| | *grated onion, fresh* |
| *1* | *tbs cider vinegar* |
| | *special boiled mayonnaise* |
| | *salt and pepper to taste* |

Combine warm potatoes, chives, salt, pepper, onion and vinegar. Stir well and chill. Meanwhile, mix celery and special boiled mayonnaise and chill. Combine potato and special boiled mayonnaise mixtures before serving.

### Chicken Salad

| | |
|---|---|
| *2* | *cups diced cooked chicken* |
| ½ | *cup chopped celery* |
| ½ | *cup grated, fresh onion* |
| | *special boiled mayonnaise* |
| | *salt and pepper to taste* |

Combine all ingredients and toss lightly to coat chicken with special boiled mayonnaise.

# Meats

### Special Hash

| | |
|---|---|
| 1 | green pepper, diced, fresh |
| 3 | medium onions, diced, fresh |
| 3 | tbs Crisco |
| 1½ | lbs ground beef |
| 1 | fresh tomato |
| ¾ | cup water |
| 1½ | tsp sea salt |
| ¼ | tsp pepper |
| 3 | cups chopped, cooked potatoes (about 4) |

Saute green pepper, onions, and bacon in Crisco in a large skillet until onions are transparent. Add meat and continue to cook until it is lightly browned. Combine tomato, water and seasonings, and add to meat mixture. Then add potatoes and cook until liquid is nearly evaporated, about 15 minutes, turning occasionally. Makes 4 hearty servings.

### Special Baked Chicken

| | |
|---|---|
| 2 | lbs chicken parts |
| ¼ | cup oil or melted Crisco |
| 1 | cup finely crushed potato chips (no preservatives) |
| | salt and pepper |

Preheat oven to 400 degrees. Dip chicken in oil. Drain. Sprinkle with salt and pepper and roll in crushed chips. Arrange in greased, shallow baking dish. Cover tightly with foil. Bake 45 minutes until tender. Uncover for at least 15 minutes to brown chicken. Serves 3.

### Special Meat Loaf

| | |
|---|---|
| 2 | lbs ground beef |
| ⅓ | cup Minute Tapioca |
| ½ | cup onion, finely chopped |
| 1½ | tsp sea salt |
| ¼ | tsp pepper |
| 1½ | cups fresh tomatoes, peeled, mashed |

## Meats (continued)

Combine all ingredients, mixing well. Then pack into a 9"× 5"×3" loaf pan. Bake at 350 degrees for 1 to 1¼ hours. Unmold on serving platter and slice. May be served hot or cold. Makes 6 to 8 servings.

### Beef Stew

| | |
|---|---|
| 1 | *lb beef, cut in 1-inch cubes* |
| 2 | *tbs melted Crisco or lard* |
| ¼ | *cup chopped onion* |
| 3 | *cups boiling water* |
| 1 | *tbs salt* |
| ⅛ | *tsp pepper* |
| 1 | *small bay leaf* |
| | *dash of thyme* |
| ¾ | *cup diced carrots, fresh* |
| ¾ | *cup diced potatoes* |
| 8-10 | *small white onions, fresh* |
| 1 | *cup boiling water* |
| 5 | *tbs potato starch* |

Brown beef in fat in a large saucepan. Add onion and saute until golden brown. Add 3 cups boiling water and seasonings, cover and simmer 1½ to 2 hours, or until meat is nearly tender. Add vegetables and continue cooking for 30 minutes longer, or until vegetables are done. Add 1 cup boiling water. Add a few tablespoons cold water to potato starch and mix to a paste. Add to stew. Cook and stir until slightly thickened.

### Swiss Steak

| | |
|---|---|
| 1 | *lb round steak* |
| | *potato meal* |
| 3 | *tbs Crisco or lard, melted* |
| | *chopped onion and celery* |
| | *salt and pepper to taste* |
| ½ | *cup water* |
| 1½ | *cups peeled tomatoes, fresh or home-canned* |

Dredge the steak well in potato meal seasoned with salt and pepper. Brown meat in melted Crisco or lard. Add remaining ingredients. Cover and bake at 325 degrees for 1½ hours. Makes 2 to 3 servings.

# Desserts

## Apple Crisp

| | |
|---|---|
| 4 | cups sliced cooking apples |
| 1 | tbs apple juice* |
| 1 | cup Quaker or Mother's Oats (quick or old-fashioned, uncooked) |
| ½ | cup honey |
| 1½ | tsp cinnamon |
| ½ | tsp salt |
| ¼ | cup melted lard |

Place apples in shallow baking dish. Sprinkle with lemon juice. Combine remaining ingredients; mix until crumbly. Sprinkle additional ¼ cup of melted lard over top. Bake in preheated moderate oven (375 degrees) for 30 minutes or until apples are tender. Makes 4 servings.
*No preservatives or additives.

## Fruit Juice Tapioca

| | |
|---|---|
| ¼ | cup Minute Tapioca |
| 2¼ | cups apple juice (fresh) |
| ¾ | cup honey |
| | dash of salt |

Mix all the ingredients in a saucepan and let stand 5 minutes. Cook and stir over medium heat until mixture comes to a boil. Cool 20 minutes. Then stir well and spoon into dessert dishes. Chill.

## Soy-Coconut Cookies

| | |
|---|---|
| 1 | cup soy flour |
| 1 | cup tapioca |
| ½ | cup safflower oil |
| ½ | tsp sea salt |
| 2 | tsp baking powder |
| ¾ | cup honey |
| ⅔ | cup coconut meal* |

Mix ingredients and roll out batter ¼ inch thick. Cut 1½ inch cookies. Bake at 375 degrees for 15-17 minutes.
*Obtainable at health food store.

## Desserts (continued)

### Rice-Raisin-Date Cookies

| | |
|---|---|
| *1 to 2* | *cups unsulfured raisins (health food store)* |
| *1* | *cup water* |
| *1* | *cup dates* |
| *1½* | *tsp sea salt* |
| *1½* | *cups rice flour* |
| *½* | *cup safflower oil or kosher margarine* |
| *1½* | *tsp baking powder* |

Mix ingredients. Form batter balls and flatten on an oiled cookie tin. Bake 5-7 minutes at 400 degrees.

### Does the sample *Multiple Elimination Diet* help detect all food allergies?

No, because a child could be allergic to some food included in this particular diet. Although the diet omits the major foods which might cause allergies, certain children may be allergic to oats, rice, apple, grape, soybean, tomato, white potato or chicken, for example.

### What should be done if a child eats some food "by mistake" during a dietary trial?

Let us suppose your child is on a diet which omits peanuts and chocolate. These foods were both omitted for one week and then, when your child is given peanuts to see if these cause allergies, he also accidentally eats some chocolate. This means that it will be difficult to interpret which food caused symptoms, if they reappeared. He should stop eating both foods. Then, one at a time, each food should be re-added, as specified in Part 2, to see which might cause allergies.

### How can you be entirely certain that a food is causing an allergy?

If you re-test a food three times, and each time your child has the same symptoms, it is more than coincidence. For example, if your child eats no chocolate for a week, and then after eating it for one day he wheezes and coughs, this is casual evidence. Wait one week and re-test it. If the symptoms occur again in the same sequence, this is more suggestive evidence. If a third trial is attempted another week later and the same sequence is noted, the evidence is almost conclusive. Even this type of dietary trial, however, is not infallible. An almond extract in the chocolate could be the allergenic substance.

### Does re-adding a food to which a child is allergic always cause symptoms?

No. A child may eliminate a food and have the allergic symptoms stop in a few days. If the food is not eaten for about two to six months, it is often found that, when the food is re-added to the diet, no adverse effects occur. This is not easily explained, but it is felt that the child's body in some way has changed in its ability to tolerate the food. Foods which are re-added to a child's diet relatively soon, for example, within five to 12 days, often will cause the same symptoms which disappeared when the food was not eaten. It is supposed that if a food were re-added too soon, the body would not have adequate time to make some necessary but poorly understood adjustment. Food challenges are most reliable after total fasting several days, but that requires your personal physician's supervision.

### What factors cause difficulty in interpreting the results of dietary studies?

The results are sometimes very definite and clear-cut. The child stops eating a food and the symptoms disappear in a few days and when the food is re-added the symptoms recur. What often happens, however, is that the food is omitted from the diet and the child seems somewhat better, but is not completely better because other substances, such as dust, continue to cause allergic symptoms. When the suspected food is re-added, the child seems to be somewhat worse but the change is not dramatic. This is why the food should be eaten in excess on the day it is to be re-added. Occasionally, the food must be eaten for several days before symptoms are seen.

Many times parents notice their child is definitely worse after a certain "well-liked" food is re-added and they tend to attribute the recurrence of symptoms to any number of psychologically more acceptable factors. A visit to a friend, for example, is blamed rather than the addition of milk to the diet. This is understandable, but allergic children do not improve until their parents realistically accept the fact that their entire way of living may have to be changed. It is not easy to cook if a child is allergic to milk or wheat. It is difficult for the child, parents and siblings, but at times, unfortunately, it is necessary.

# The Rotary Diet

**How and when do you use a *Rotary Diet*?**

This diet is thought to aid in the detection of major food offenders and to help prevent the development of new food problems. It is especially helpful for infants who eat only a few foods or for children and adults who have multiple food sensitivities.

A different group of foods is eaten for each of four days and then the cycle is repeated. You can select as many of the foods allowed on a specific day as you like, but it is essential that no food be ingested more often than every four days.

Most patients do not improve for about 12 to 16 days after the *Rotary Diet* is begun. If a food is a health problem, it will be detected readily because exaggerated symptoms often occur within an hour after that food is eaten. If the same food item causes symptoms every four days, it is easy to spot the one causing symptoms.

If a breast-fed infant has allergic symptoms, the mother should try a *Rotary Diet*. Foods which the mother eats pass readily into her milk.

Colic, irritability, hives, skin rash, insomnia or asthma can occur shortly after an infant is breast-fed milk which contains a food to which the baby is sensitive. Mothers worry that they cannot produce milk if milk and dairy products are not ingested. The healthy body can produce milk from other foods.

**Are there special tips for the *Rotary Diet*?**
1. This kind of a diet requires planning and determination. It is very difficult at first, but once you have carried it out for about 12 days it becomes easier to plan your menus.
2. Read *all* the fine print on *all* food labels.
3. During the first four to eight days of the diet, eat only the foods which you believe to be no problem.
4. At first, start with a few of each day's allowed foods and if your child remains well, gradually expand the number of foods eaten on each day of the four-day cycle. Add new foods one at a time once you find that no health problems are noted on a certain day of the cycle.
5. You can switch a food from one day to another day if you have some special preferences. Once you have made this decision, try to maintain a consistent schedule. Always keep chicken and egg on the same day; the same applies for beef and milk.

6. If you switch a food from one day to another, all the foods listed in parentheses go with that food because they are all botanically related (see *Rotary Diet* Schedule, pp. 170–173). For example, you can't have orange one day, lemon the next and grapefruit on the third. They are all citrus, and sensitivity to one often means sensitivity to the rest.

7. If you find there is not enough to eat on a particular day of the four-day cycle, move some food from a day which has too many foods to a day which has too few. Learn to eat foods which you have not eaten before. Obtain some helpful books which have recipes and suggestions for this type of diet. You must develop some ingenuity.

8. Put fruit, glass-bottled spring water and the sweetener of the day in a blender to make a beverage to drink and use on cereal. If fruit causes diarrhea, use more water and less fruit.

9. Make a soup for each day with the allowed meat and vegetables for that day. Store the excess in *glass* jars in the freezer until the next time that day of the cycle recurs. Buy no soups, as most have additives.

10. Use *fresh* fruits, vegetables and meats. Organically grown ones are best but may not be available in many areas of the country. Eat no luncheon meats, sausage, ham, bacon, fresh-frozen or pre-packaged foods with dyes, additives or preservatives.

11. Use sea salt. This is available from health food stores.

12. If milk and soymilk are not tolerated, check with your physician about a calcium substitute to help ensure normal bone growth.

13. If the patient is sick repeatedly on a certain day of the four-day cycle, he should try to eat each food for that day separately, allowing an hour or so between each one, throughout the entire day. This allows for easy detection of the offending food item. Watch for a possible pulse increase of 20 or more points after a test food is eaten. This sometimes happens. It often indicates that a problem food has been found.

14. Continue this diet for weeks or months if it keeps your child well and healthy. Be certain your physician approves of a prolonged diet from the nutrition viewpoint.

# RECORDS FOR A ROTARY DIET

Rotary Diet

Name

| Date | Record EVERYTHING EATEN each day. | | | | Record in RED when symptoms begin on any day. | | | |
|---|---|---|---|---|---|---|---|---|
| | Day 1 | Day 2 | Day 3 | Day 4 | Day 1 | Day 2 | Day 3 | Day 4 |
| BREAKFAST | | | | | | | | |
| SNACKS | | | | | | | | |
| LUNCH | | | | | | | | |
| SNACKS | | | | | | | | |

DINNER

SNACKS

MISCELLANEOUS

Used by permission of Syntex Laboratories. From the booklet *Food Sensitivity Diets*. © 1978 by Doris J. Rapp.

SAMPLE

### Rotary Diet for Infants

Start with 1 or 2 foods each day. Add more single foods as needed.

| Days 1, 5, 9, etc. | Days 2, 6, 10, etc. | Days 3, 7, 11, etc. | Days 4, 8, 12, etc. |
|---|---|---|---|
| cow's milk | diluted orange juice | soy milk | diluted grape juice |
| wheat | rice | oats | barley |

Later on, add in manner indicated below

| | | | |
|---|---|---|---|
| squash | carrots | string beans | white potato |
| peach + juice | pineapple + juice | apple sauce + apple juice | banana + water (blender) |
| beef | tuna | chicken | lamb |

*Rotary Diet* for **Children and Adults**

|  | Days 1,5,9, etc. | Days 2,6,10, etc. | Days 3,7,11, etc. | Days 4,8,12, etc. |
|---|---|---|---|---|
| Grains and Cereals | Wheat cereal (macaroni and noodles, if eggs allowed) | Corn cereal (bread, muffins—canned or fresh) Millet* | Rice cereal or rice Rykrisp Rye bread (Bread of Life)* | Barley—cereal or grain Oats—cereal or baked Poi, taro* |
| Fruits, Fresh Juice, Jelly | Apple (pear) Figs (mulberry) | Cranberry (blueberry, wintergreen, hazelnut) Plums (prunes, peaches, apricots, cherries, almonds) | Grapes (raisins) Pineapple Elderberry Currants (gooseberry) Orange (grapefruit, tangerine, lemon, lime) | Blackberry (raspberry, boysenberry, strawberry)* Banana |
| Vegetables | Carrots (celery, dill, parsnip, parsley) Lettuce (artichoke, endive) Beets (spinach) | Asparagus (onions, chives, leeks, garlic) Cabbage (brussels sprouts, broccoli, cauliflower, turnip, mustard) | White potatoes (any form), potato chips, tomato, eggplant, String beans (lima beans, navy beans, peanuts, peas, soybeans, licorice) | Sweet potatoes (any form) Cucumbers (pickles, squash, melon, watermelon, pumpkin, cantaloupe) |

* Can be purchased at most health food stores.

*Rotary Diet* for Children and Adults (cont.)

| | Days 1,5,9, etc. | Days 2,6,10, etc. | Days 3,7,11, etc. | Days 4, 8, 12, etc. |
|---|---|---|---|---|
| Meats or Fish | Chicken (turkey, pheasant) | Lamb or add ONE of the following:<br>1. tuna<br>2. scallops (oysters, clams)<br>3. salmon (trout, whitefish)<br>4. shrimp (lobster, crab)<br>5. whitefish<br>6. cod<br>7. pike<br>8. perch<br>9. halibut (sole, flounder) | Pork | Beef<br>Duck or goose<br>Rabbit |
| Snacks | Olives (black, green)<br>Cashews (pistachios)<br>Chestnuts | Brazil nuts<br>Popcorn (and Crisco oil or corn oil)<br>Coconut (and oil) | Filberts<br>Hazel nuts | Walnuts<br>Pecans |

|  | Days 1,5,9, etc. | Days 2,6,10, etc. | Days 3,7,11, etc. | Days 4, 8, 12, etc. |
|---|---|---|---|---|
| Spices and Miscellaneous | Avocado (cinnamon, bay leaf) Apple cider vinegar Peppermint (spearmint, basil, marjoram, sage, savory, thyme) Cottonseed oil (Wesson) Eggs Yeast Olive oil Beet sugar | Dates (coconut) Date sugar Karo syrup Corn oil (Mazola) Corn sugar Corn syrup | Mushrooms Soy oil* or peanut oil Soybean milk ice cream (flavored with chocolate, carob, honey, pineapple or orange) Yeast Honey Cara-Coa soy candy* | Sunflower seeds Safflower oil* Cottage cheese Butter Vanilla ice cream Walnuts and pecans Maple syrup (pure) Maple sugar (pure) Yogurt Cane sugar |
| Beverages | See juices above Comfrey tea | See juices above Papaya Kaffir tea | Tea—plain or orange-flavored Coffee Rich Dark chocolate (cocoa) Cola | Coffee Milk |

* Can be purchased at most health food stores.

Used by permission of Syntex Laboratories. From the booklet *Food Sensitivity Diets.* © 1978 by Doris J. Rapp.

## SPECIAL PROBLEMS RELATED TO CERTAIN FOODS

### Will older children drink soybean milk?

Often they will not. It helps if it is mixed as directed on the can and placed into a very clean container. When it is chilled it tastes very similar to milk. Try giving it on cereal first. Soybean milk causes bowel movements to become softer than normal.

### How can you make ice cream using soybean milk?

Soybean milk ice cream (which does not contain regular milk but could cause symptoms in patients sensitive to sugar, corn or pork) can be made in the following manner:[1]

### REFRIGERATOR TRAY METHOD

*1 13-oz. can Isomil concentrate, well chilled (do not dilute with water).*

*1½ teaspoons unflavored gelatin. Soften in 2 tablespoons cold water.*

*¼ cup sugar. Add to the gelatin and heat slowly to dissolve sugar and gelatin; cool.*

*2 tablespoons clear corn syrup.*

*1 tablespoon salad/cooking oil (e.g., A & P Dexola soybean oil).*

*2 teaspoons vanilla extract*

*Add fresh blended or pureed fruit if it does not cause allergy.*

Blend all ingredients[2] in a blender until thick and creamy. Pour into an ice cube tray or a loaf pan and freeze until very icy. Turn into blender and blend until smooth. Return to freezer and freeze until firm. Allow to soften slightly before serving. Blender capacity for this recipe should be at least 5 cups.

---

[1] Acknowledgment and special thanks for recipe development to Dr. Merle S. Scherr, Medical Director, and Mrs. Nancy G. Altman, Consultant Research Dietitian, Bronco Junction Summer Camp for Asthmatic Children, Allergy Rehabilitation Foundation, Inc., Charleston, West Virginia. Acknowledgment is due to Ross Laboratories, a division of Abbott Laboratories, Columbus, Ohio, for permission to include this recipe.

[2] Individual flavor variations: fruits such as strawberries, peaches, bananas, pineapples, oranges, etc., may be added to recipe prior to freezing after being mashed or pureed in a blender, depending upon individual tastes and allergies. Avoid artificially colored fruits.

**If your child has a possible milk, wheat or egg allergy, how can these foods be avoided in all forms?**

Learn which foods contain these substances. Read all product labels and avoid any foods in which the ingredients are not listed. (Refer to Appendix II.) Have your child eat mainly meat, fruit and vegetables.

**Is food labeling accurate?**

Usually it is, but at times it is misleading. For example, a product which contains milk may state only that it contains sodium caseinate. The latter is a milk product. Some products which contain a small amount of sodium caseinate are clearly labeled "milk-free." This is not true, and someone highly allergic to milk could have symptoms from eating such a product.

Foods may not state that they contain eggs, but rather may list that they contain vitellin or ovovitellin, livetin, ovomucoid, ovomucin, albumin or globulin. These are all egg proteins and could conceivably cause allergies.

**What is the relationship between an allergy to female chicken and eggs?**

There are definitely some children who are allergic to both. Interestingly, however, some egg-allergic patients can eat male chicken (such as a capon or rooster) without difficulty. It is felt that the female, or hen, chicken's meat possibly has some protein in common with eggs or that it is contaminated by the eggs produced, thus causing a reaction to both. The explanation and scientific verification of this occurrence is inadequate.

**What is the relationship between allergies to milk and to beef?**

Such a sensitivity can and does occur. The beef allergy is usually less frequent and severe than the milk sensitivity.

**What bread substitutes are available?**

Canned rye bread and a type of rice biscuit which do not contain wheat are available. Toasting this special rye bread enhances its flavor. Some health food stores carry these products, or you may write directly to the supplier.

Most readily purchased breads, including rye, rice, potato and gluten, contain wheat. It is very difficult to bake bread without using some wheat flour.

**Where can flour which is made from pure rye, potatoes, oats or barley be purchased?**

From a health food store. Check the Yellow Pages of any telephone directory.

**How can you make gravy without wheat flour?**

Use arrowroot. This seldom causes allergy. Cornstarch can cause allergies if a child is allergic to corn; the same is true of potato starch.

**Are there any special precautions for children who are allergic to fish?**

Children who cannot eat fish often cannot tolerate the smell of fish. Such children could possibly have difficulty in school cafeterias or restaurants serving fish, or in meat markets or stores selling fish. Pizza with anchovies, clam chowder or certain fish-type chip dips could also be troublesome. Glue that is caramel colored may be made from fish. Old books which have glue in the binding could cause symptoms. Stamp collections, stamps, or photo-mounting hinges could cause difficulty. Cleaning fishtanks or fishing can be a problem. Cod liver oil tablets or capsules should never be taken by such children.

**Are there any special precautions related to citrus fruit allergy?**

Some children are sensitive to only one of the citrus fruits but others could have symptoms from oranges, grapefruits, lemons, limes, tangerines or kumquats. Juices, soda pop, Kool-Aid, Jell-O, candy (such as suckers or sour balls) and certain medicines, lozenges or cough drops could contain citrus fruit flavor and cause allergic problems in some children. Alka-Seltzer Antacid Formula (in gold foil) contains citric acid.

**What can a child eat as a chocolate substitute?**

Colored or white chocolate is as allergenic as ordinary chocolate. There is a form of chocolate made from soybeans which is sold in health food stores. There is a second type called Cara-Coa made from carob.

**Is food storage a problem?**

Some patients cannot tolerate food stored in plastic containers because the plastic residue seeps into the food. The phenolic lining in food cans may also affect the phenol- (Lysol-) sensitive patient. The corn in some milk containers can be a problem for corn-sensitive patients. Use glass containers wherever possible. Canned potato chips (without additives) can cause difficulties in some patients because of the gas used to retain the product's freshness. Even the chemicals in the clear paper used to wrap meat or cover refrigerated foods can cause symptoms. Storage in glass containers is best.

## OTHER MEDICAL PROBLEMS WHICH MIGHT BE RELATED TO FOOD ALLERGIES

**What are cold sores?**

Cold sores (herpes simplex) are small water blisters which frequently form along the edge of the lips. Sunlight and irritation are believed to activate a dormant virus in that area, causing cold sore eruption in some people.

**Are cold sores related to food allergies?**

Yes. In particular fresh fruits, chocolate, peppermint or gum seem to activate the virus causing cold sores. Keep a diary of the unusual foods eaten for the 24-hour period *before* the cold sore starts and subsequently check each food by not eating it for a week and then eating it in excess for three days (in addition to your usual diet) to see if it truly causes a cold sore. There are many cases where allergies are not found to be the responsible factor. Many times the cause of this problem is never determined. A promising new treatment using dilutions of flu vaccine is being investigated at present.

**What are canker sores?**

These are rounded, painful, open sores usually located on the inside of the cheek or gums, near the teeth. At times these are felt to be related to exposure to citrus fruits in some form (fresh and frozen juices, candy, Popsicles™ or Jell-O) or by contact with acetic acid (vinegar). The offending item is often eaten about eight hours before the first sores are noted.

**Can migraine headaches be caused by allergy?**

Yes. These are frequently one-sided and located near the temple in the area of the forehead between the eye and the ear. These occur more often in women and are frequently preceded by visual problems, paleness or weakness. They are often associated with an emotional upset and nausea, or abdominal discomfort. These headaches are noted for their intense severity, duration for hours or days and poor response to aspirin. Many allergic families include members who have this problem. Children are most apt to have this form of allergy after puberty, but it is often difficult for very young children to say that they have a headache.

Common allergy-related causes of migraines are milk (cheese), chocolate (cola), corn, eggs, peas, peanuts, cinnamon, oregano, garlic, pork, molds, dust, pollens and pets. Triggering factors can be tobacco smoke, odors, emotional upsets, fatigue, chilling, hunger and menses.

Drugs are commonly used to treat migraines and, *if* allergy is a factor, antihistamines, avoidance diets and allergy extracts might prove helpful. Osteopathic adjustments help some patients. Many chronic headaches and migraines are related to a sensitivity to a number of foods, pollens or molds, dust, chemical fumes, natural gas heat or hormones. Stress aggravates or precipitates the onset unless the basic causes are eliminated or avoided whenever possible.

### What is the allergic-tension fatigue syndrome?

People who feel tense or who are hyperactive, convulsive, generally fatigued, drowsy or lethargic, or who have muscle and joint aches, vague fevers and mild to severe behavior and learning disorders may not know that *sometimes* these problems can be due to allergy. Eating certain foods, drinking tap water or contact with items such as dust, pets, perfume, tobacco, odorous plastics, aerosols or insecticides have caused such symptoms. Until more research can be done to study this type of nervous system allergy, we must be satisfied in knowing that the elimination of the causative factor apparently relieves some patients' symptoms.

### Do megavitamins and special nutrition diets help allergy?

Some physicians and nutrition specialists claim that they do. They believe that vitamins and diets alter the bodies of certain people so they may be less prone to develop allergies to things that don't affect most persons. The use of trace metals and minerals, as well as large doses of many B-complex vitamins and Vitamin C, may prove to be another avenue of help, particularly for patients (such as hyperactive children) who have nervous system allergy. The effectiveness of such therapy is not fully documented scientifically at the present time, but a gradual increase of clinical and research evidence is beginning to accumulate to confirm the initial impressions.

# PART FOUR

# How your physician does allergy testing and treatment

CHAPTER 10 includes many details concerning one common method of detecting allergies using tests done on or in the skin. From the interpretation of these skin tests and the patient's history, a special medicine called an allergy extract is often prepared.

˙Chapter 11 tells what is and is not contained in such extracts and how and where they are injected. It is essential that any patient receiving such therapy understand what normally happens and should not happen after an allergy-extract injection. It explains when you should or should not receive such treatments. Some clues are given as to how a physician decides when this form of therapy can be stopped.

# CHAPTER 10

# *Skin testing*

**What are allergy skin tests?**

Tests which are done on or in the skin to determine the cause of allergies are known as skin tests. Other tests which might be done on rare occasion would include having the child breathe certain substances into the lungs or by placing certain allergenic substances in the eyes or nose or under the tongue (sublingual tests).

**What are the usual types of skin tests and how are they done?**

There are a number of ways to skin test for allergy. The first are the *traditional* ones, which are accepted by most allergists although each has his personal preferences. Some use only scratch or prick tests, others use only intradermal or needle tests, and many use both types. There is no doubt that many patients are helped by treatment based on the results of these accepted tests. Intradermal testing is often done first with a weak, and later with a strong, extract solution of the items in question.

A newer method of testing uses a number of skin tests for each allergenic substance which is to be checked. The patient is tested with a strong solution and later with weaker solutions. It is often found that the strong solution will produce mild, typical symptoms, while a weaker solution causes the patient's symptoms to subside. Treatment with an allergy extract medicine which contains the exact dilution which eliminated the patient's symptoms during testing is sometimes very effective.

These newer methods are presently under careful scrutiny to evaluate their efficacy. Although scientific documentation is not available as yet, these newer methods show great promise in providing more specific answers to the exact causes of many types of specific allergy symptoms.

In general, the weaker the extract-testing solution needed to cause a reaction, the more sensitive the child. Stronger, larger, more itchy reactions often denote a greater sensitivity or allergy.

## What is a typical reaction to an allergy skin test?

The most common reaction, if someone is allergic to a substance, is a local hive or mosquito bite-like swelling at the site or area of the skin test. This is called an immediate skin-test reaction and usually occurs in about ten minutes and lasts about 30 minutes or less. This can cause slight itching but is rarely severe. If a child is not allergic to the testing material, the skin in the area of the test appears entirely normal after about ten minutes. At times, there is no immediate reaction to a skin test but the next day there might be a red, itchy area about one-quarter to one-half inch in diameter which gradually subsides or disappears during the next couple of days. This is a delayed skin reaction and should be reported to your allergist, as it may indicate a significant allergy.

## Can skin tests cause sudden, alarming allergic symptoms?

Yes, but only on rare occasions. Intradermal or possibly scratch tests could cause asthma or hay fever if the child had an *exquisite* sensitivity to such substances as cats, dogs, horses, eggs, fish, nuts, cottonseed, mustard or glue. Parents would, however, usually know about such extreme allergies and there would be no need to test for substances which obviously cause difficulty. Mild allergic reactions can occur during testing.

Some allergists routinely test with food or pollen extracts of varying strengths in order to produce mild to moderate symptoms. This is called a provocation test and tends to confirm that the test item does produce a specific symptom.

## How many skin tests are usually done for a complete allergic evaluation?

This would vary greatly from child to child and depend upon the symptoms and severity of the allergy. There are many justifiable variables plus personal preferences, but roughly from 20 to 100 scratch tests and 50 to 200 intradermal tests might be done.

Titration testing might entail as many as 120 tests for 30 allergic substances.

## How many skin tests are done in one visit?

It would vary with the age and size of the child. Usually five to 30 intradermal skin tests are done per office visit or about 20 or 30 scratch tests. Titration testing requires visits which last three hours or so. At least one item would be tested each ten minutes.

**If a child's allergic problems occur only during a few selected weeks each year, would complete allergy testing be needed?**

No. Usually tests would be carried out only for those substances most apt to cause trouble at the time of year when symptoms were noted. For example, symptoms occurring for only one week in April would probably be due to tree allergies and testing would be needed for only the few trees which might cause symptoms during that particular week. Symptoms in July could be due to grass pollens, mold spores or both, and tests for these only would be indicated if the symptoms only occurred at this time. It is unnecessary to test for summer grass allergy if the patient's symptoms occur only in winter.

**Do skin tests hurt?**

The scratch or prick tests usually tickle. The intradermal tests hurt about as much as a fingernail pressed into the skin or a slight pinch.

Most children over four or five can be tested without difficulty or obvious discomfort. Children under four are a challenge because they often cry before testing is even attempted. Most children do not fear the tests and many actually look forward to their visits. Some who are fearful of needles prior to the visit to the allergist learn that they are not painful and subsequently are not afraid. Some children at any age, especially if they were frightened during medical treatment in the past, are most difficult. Parents can help greatly to give their child assurance. The office visit should not be mentioned until the time of the visit so that children who do worry won't think about it for days in advance. Explain that the test feels like a slight prick or sharp fingernail and that they must make their parents proud. Occasionally, a mother's actions can make her child fearful.

**Are skin tests always reliable?**

No. Certain drugs such as antihistamines, if taken shortly before skin testing is performed, could make it very difficult to interpret the test reactions.

A positive skin test cannot be evaluated unless the physician has been given a detailed history concerning the child's allergies.

At times a skin test reflects a past allergy. For example, an infant might be allergic to eggs and "outgrow" this allergy yet still have a positive skin-test reaction to eggs when adulthood is reached. At other times a skin test shows or predicts a future allergy. It is not unusual to find a child who has a positive skin reaction to ragweed and has never had obvious allergic symptoms at the time of the year when ragweed is in the air. This type of child often develops corresponding symptoms within two or more years of the time when the positive skin test is noted.

Usually, however, a positive skin-test reaction means that the patient is presently allergic to the substance used for skin testing. If there is doubt, the skin test can be confirmed by a clinical trial, such as eating the food in question at an interval of five days, or by inhaling or breathing a substance which is suspected of causing the allergy. This type of trial should be carried out only under the supervision of your physician since it could be dangerous if done incorrectly.

Of all the allergy skin tests performed, those involving food sensitivity are the most unreliable, inasmuch as food-testing extracts are not stable (especially certain fresh fruits or vegetables) and because cooking and digestion changes foods to such a great degree that they are not the same as the food extract usually used for skin testing. Some foods which elicit no skin reaction may in fact produce allergies because cooking and digestion changes them into a form that causes a reaction inside the body. Newer, serial titration testing, performed with strong and weak food extracts, more accurately detects offending foods by provoking mild symptoms during the test procedures.

### Is it possible for a child to be allergic to some substance which caused no reaction on skin testing?

Yes, this sometimes happens. Although the skin-test reaction is entirely negative, pollen, for example, when placed in the eye or nose or breathed into the lungs, can cause symptoms. Such patients may respond well to pollen-extract therapy. Titration testing also does not always cause symptoms but changes in the skin-test reaction can indicate an allergy.

### Can a child be allergic to a food which he has never eaten?

It is possible for a child to have a positive skin-test reaction to a certain food and to other foods in the same class or category (see Appendix II), although the latter may never have been eaten. For example, a patient allergic to orange could also be allergic to lime or lemon. All are citrus fruits and a patient can be allergic to the same component which is found in all of them. This explains why children who can't eat shrimp often have similar symptoms when eating lobster, which is also a crustacean. The skin reaction to both would often be positive, although only one had been eaten in the past. However, an allergy to one food in a category does not necessarily signify an allergy to all foods in that class. Peanuts, peas and string beans are all legumes. Frequently, children are seen who have severe allergies from eating peanuts, mild symptoms from peas and no difficulty at all with beans.

Breast milk contains what the mother eats and some infants develop food allergy from the foods forming breast milk.

### Can a child's allergy tests be performed in his parent's skin rather than his own?

Yes, this is possible but the skin tests would not be as reliable as direct testing on a patient's own skin. The skin tests do not cause enough discomfort to warrant this procedure except under most exceptional circumstances. Most young children need few skin tests and older children almost never object.

### Do all children need skin tests?

No. At times the allergist can determine exactly what is causing the problem entirely from the history of when and where the child has symptoms. It could be a food, a feather or kapok pillow or a household pet. Elimination of the offending substance may solve the problem. To be entirely certain, it sometimes helps to eliminate a potential cause of difficulty to see if the problem subsides or stops, then to expose the child again to see if symptoms recur. This should not be done if exposure causes serious symptoms. If, however, a child seems to be allergic to many substances, skin testing may have to be carried out. As many as 80 to 90 per cent of children seeing an allergist may need skin testing.

### May medicines be taken before skin testing?

It depends on the medicine. Aspirin, antibiotics, or cortisone (steroids) do not affect a skin test. Most drugs used to treat hay fever, asthma, or allergies and some cough medicines might alter skin-test reactions, so these should be avoided preferably for 24 hours (at least 8 to 12) before tests.

### What do you do when a child wheezes on the day when skin-testing is scheduled?

If the wheeze is severe, give asthma medicine and call the doctor. No testing can be done on a child who is having a severe asthma attack, but the doctor may have to see your child to treat the acute wheezing episode.

If the wheeze is moderate or slight, call your physician and ask if the tests can be done just *before* a dose of medicine is due. The allergy medicines can be given ten minutes after testing.

## Do skin tests ever have to be repeated?

Yes. It is very possible for a child to become allergic to a new substance to which he may be exposed. If a child who has been well on allergy treatment begins to have allergic symptoms again, this often means something "new" is now affecting him; if his history does not reveal the offending agent, additional tests may have to be done.

Children in the two-to-five-year age group, in particular, are apt to develop new allergies and might need selected or complete retesting as they become older.

## What does the allergist do after the skin tests are completed?

A careful evaluation of your child's history, physical examination, other laboratory studies and skin tests is made. The allergist may then make recommendations concerning your child's home, environment and diet. If indicated, a special extract or several extracts may be prepared. These would contain various substances to which your child was allergic and for which the physician felt your child should be treated. Some substances can be avoided, but not completely, and treatments with extracts are usually needed for these. All substances which cause skin reactions cannot be placed into extracts. For example, wool is seldom used in extract medicines. Various pollens may be placed in one extract and other substances (such as dust), which cause mainly winter allergies, might be placed in another.

Food-extract therapy is presently used by a growing minority of allergists. Preliminary research indicates this may be a new adjunct in food therapy.

## Can a blood test replace skin tests for allergy?

New blood serum tests for total immunoglobulin E often can indicate if allergy is present in infants, children and adults. A RAST test for specific allergens such as dust and pollen is as reliable as a skin test. RAST tests detect some foods which cause immediate reactions when they are eaten but do *not* detect the more common food reactions which occur several hours after ingestion. Bioassay serial titration food testing is more reliable for these food problems.

## Do hospital evaluations help?

There is little doubt that individual food challenges after a four- to six-day water fast is the most reliable method to determine exactly what effect a food (or chemical exposure) has on a patient's health. Only a few hospitals in the U.S.A. presently have a truly allergy-free environment in which to do this type of testing. Such studies quickly eliminate a patient's symptoms due to foods, chemicals or the environment. The problem is that, although a definitive diagnosis is made as to the cause of the medical problem, specific therapy or avoidance may create a major and costly challenge in day-to-day living.

**What tests, other than allergy skin tests, might an allergist do?**

There are several, depending upon the type of allergy a patient has.

For chest allergies, a chest X-ray and test for tuberculosis (or possibly other infectious diseases) are needed. For allergies of the nose or ears, sinus X-rays are often necessary. An X-ray to determine the size of the adenoids might also be indicated.

A blood examination is often required to determine the number of "allergic-type" white blood cells, called eosinophils, which are in the blood. Nose, eye, ear, chest or stool mucus is also often examined to determine if it contains an excess of eosinophils. If these cells predominate, it usually means that the patient has allergies. In certain selected children, other tests, such as those which evaluate breathing or lung function, might be advisable.

Some children who have excessive infections associated with allergies might need special gamma- or other globulin determinations. Your physician will decide exactly which tests are necessary for your child.

# CHAPTER 11

# *Allergy-extract treatments*

On the following pages, unless otherwise specified, all statements related to allergy-extract treatment medicine refer to the aqueous or "water" form rather than to the various other longer-acting types of extracts (such as Allpyral) used to treat allergies.

There are two general methods of treatment with aqueous allergy extract.

1. The *traditional method*, which has changed little in the past 50 years and is used and accepted by most allergists.

2. The newer method, using a *bioassay titration end-point*, which is controversial. Although the results of several large scientific studies presently in progress to evaluate its efficacy are not available, a small but growing number of allergists are now trying and accepting this method.

Both methods have skeptics who feel that neither is helpful. Both methods cause similar changes in the blood of treated patients, but these changes may show no relationship to the degree of improvement which a patient notices. In the final analysis only one thing really counts. Is the patient helped without being harmed?

## Do allergy-extract treatments really help most children who have allergies?

Yes. Most are helped. About 80 per cent of those children treated for pollen sensitivity improve. If a child is being cared for by a well trained allergist, improvement is usually, but not always, noted. In some instances, the parents of an allergic child and the allergist do everything possible to help the child improve, yet problems persist. This, fortunately, is rare. There are also instances when the physician and parent know why the child's problems continue but because of some unfortunate, extenuating circumstance the problem cannot be eliminated. An example would be a mother with ten children living in a 100-year-old house. To make and to keep a room "allergy-free" under such circumstances would be almost impossible.

In other children, the allergy problem continues because the family refuses to part with a loved pet or the child insists on eating "just a little" of the food causing the asthma or nasal allergies.

### How long must a child receive allergy-injection treatments before improvement is noted?

There are marked individual differences. Once *traditional* allergy-extract treatments are started, a fortunate child may be using less medicine and have fewer symptoms in a couple of months, but it generally takes about six to eight months before obvious improvement is noted. An occasional child may not improve for one or two years. If a child is responding favorably to treatment, the child should have fewer symptoms and be using less medicine as time passes. Each year, taken as a whole, should be better than the previous year.

The newer *bioassay titration* method of determining the treatment dosage of allergy extracts enables the "correct" individualized dosage to be determined within an hour after testing and improvement can be evident in one day to two weeks. These newer methods need further scientific documentation.

### How is a child treated with an allergy extract?

In *traditional* allergy treatment, the child is started initially on injections of allergenic substances which are highly diluted. The dosage and strength of the extract is raised to a top level (usual top dosage is 0.5 to 1 cc, or one-eighth to one-quarter of a teaspoon). This is a level which affords adequate protection to most patients. Some children respond well to lower-than-average doses of extracts and these patients can be maintained on less potent extract. The injections cause changes so that exposure to previously troublesome allergens produces less difficulty. The fact that allergists cannot explain to their entire satisfaction exactly why patients improve when given extract treatments in no way detracts from the fact that such treatments do help.

The newer, controversial *titration* methods of treatment entail no or very few "build-up" injections. Treatments with the "correct" dose are taken as needed every few hours or days. Whenever symptoms are noted, more treatment is given and the symptoms often subside within minutes. The treatments can be given under the tongue (sublingual) as extract drops or by injection. Injection therapy gives relief more quickly and for a longer period of time than sublingual therapy. However, the latter has obvious advantages.

## How often does a child need to receive an allergy-injection treatment?

With *traditional* allergy-extract treatment, a child initially receives injections of the extract medicine one to three times a week.

The number of so-called "build-up" injections required until the top dosage is reached may vary from 10 to 40. This build-up of the strength or amount of the extract medicine requires visits to the physician at frequent intervals (one to three times weekly).

For example, the first treatment consists of a small amount of a "weak" extract medicine, the next a larger amount of the same and gradually, as more injections are administered, the child would start to be given a small amount of "strong" extract. Finally the object is to increase the amount and strength to what is best for a particular child. This is called the "top-tolerated dosage" and amounts to about five to ten drops. Once this dosage is reached, treatments are needed and given only once every four to five weeks for a period of roughly five to twenty or more years. Select patients may need routine treatments more often or extra booster injections during a pollen season.

The newer titration end-point method enables the patient to treat himself either with drops under the tongue or by injection. The drops are initially used three times or so daily, but after a few weeks twice a day suffices and after a few months many require treatment only once or twice a week. The same dosage can be administered by injection, usually once daily at first, but later once or twice a week. When symptoms recur, the "correct" dosage is administered and the patient's symptoms should subside within a few minutes without other medication. If they do not, an adjustment must be made in the "correct" dosage. During the pollen season, treatments may be needed on a daily basis. Patients with year-round problems need extra treatments only if exposed to an excessive amount of the item to which they are sensitive.

## How important is it to receive *traditional* allergy-injection treatments on the exact date they are due to be given?

The answer would vary according to certain specific circumstances. In general, extracts usually can be given on a date *earlier* than when a child is due to receive them. This is sometimes necessary when a child is going on a trip or leaving town.

1. *For Children Just Beginning Extract Treatments*—If a child is just beginning to receive injection treatments and is due to see the physician two or three times a week, it is not essential that every appointment be kept. Missed appointments, however, mean that it will take more time before a child improves.

2. *For Children on a Four- or Five-Week Schedule*—It is most essential that the allergy-extract injections never be given at more than a 35-day interval. If the interval of time between the treatments is longer than this, there is a possibility that if the previous dose of extract were repeated, it might cause an allergic reaction. To be safe, your physician will have to lower the dosage if the interval between the injection treatments is too great, and additional visits would be required before the dosage could be re-raised to the previous customary maximum level.

3. *For Children Who Are Having Their Extract Dosage Re-raised*—If a child for some reason is having his extract-dosage level raised, he will need injections every 14 days. If the interval of time between treatments is greater than this, the dosage cannot be increased.

### What is usually included in extracts used to treat allergies?

Traditionally, a child may be treated with single substances which cause allergy or several substances combined into one or two extracts. Extracts frequently contain dust, feathers, kapok, cotton linters, mold spores, tree, grass and weed pollens. At times, if excessive infections are a problem, a bacterial vaccine might be included, although this form of therapy is controversial.

The newer *titration end-point* therapy includes the same allergenic items, except that foods and animal dander are often included in the treatment extract. It is difficult to treat for chemical pollutants of many types. Avoidance of these items is a major therapeutic challenge.

### What is usually not put into an allergy extract?

*Traditional* allergy extract excludes foods, insecticides, cottonseed, flaxseed, silk, wool, and animal danders (see Chapter 15). These substances can often be avoided.

### What location on the arm should be used for extract injections?

There is no location which is really best. It is a matter of the physician's or patient's personal preference. The injections should be given low enough on the arm that a tourniquet could be applied if the patient had a reaction to the injection. The treatments can be given into one arm on one visit and into the other on the next. Occasionally, if a child repeatedly has uncomfortable reactions in the area of the injection, merely changing the location of the treatment eliminates this problem. Discuss this possibility with the physician giving the injections.

### What is a "normal" reaction to a *traditional* allergy-extract injection treatment?

Usually the skin in the area of the injection appears entirely normal or a small area of redness, itching or swelling may occur. This area may be about one or one and one-half inches in diameter and one-quarter inch thick or less and it should not be swollen for longer than 24 hours. Occasionally the site is sore but there is little or no redness, and this may last for one or two days. If the site is painful, do not massage it. When the child is initially receiving weak extract medicine, there is no or only a slight local reaction. If a marked local reaction is noted, check with your allergist. As a patient is approaching the maximum strength of extract that can be received, a slight local reaction frequently occurs. It is not abnormal for the site of an allergy injection to hurt if accidentally bumped. This can occur during sleep, in particular.

Bioassay titration end-point injection therapy usually causes no local swelling or redness.

### What is a mild, "abnormal," local reaction to a traditional allergy-extract treatment?

If the swelling or pain in the area of the extract treatment is so great that the arm hurts when the patient is dressing or writing, the reaction is too great. It is not normal for the swelling to be so large that it extends from the shoulder to the elbow.

The arm should not hurt for more than one and one-half days after a treatment. If this occurs, discuss it with your allergist.

Abnormal reactions to the newer titration end-point therapy indicate the need for an adjustment in the therapeutic dose.

### What abnormal reactions can occur from allergy-injection treatments which are not localized in the injection area?

Any of the following can possibly occur in any sequence or combination. The intensity of any of these symptoms can range from very mild to extremely severe. None of the following, *even in a mild form,* should *suddenly* become evident within two hours after an allergy treatment is given:

| | |
|---|---|
| stuffiness of the nose | red ear lobes |
| itching of the nose or throat | shortness of breath |
| sneezing | difficult breathing or asthma |
| tearing of the eyes | headache |
| itching of the eyes | hoarseness |

| | |
|---|---|
| throat-clearing | abdominal pain, diarrhea |
| swelling of lips | or vomiting |
| coughing | uterine contractions or |
| | vaginal bleeding |

hives or itchy skin[1] (especially in the arm creases near the elbow, or in the palms)

If an unusual reaction occurs after an injection of the "correct" dosage determined by titration end-point, no further therapy can be administered until appropriate adjustment is made. An alarming reaction to this type of therapy would be most unusual.

## What should you do about a reaction to an allergy-extract treatment?

For a normal or mild abnormal local reaction do the following:

1. If the area of the injection hurts, give aspirin or an aspirin substitute. The dose of aspirin for children is one grain for each year of age up to the age of five. This can be repeated in four hours. For example, a five-year-old could be given five grains every four hours. Aspirin tablets are available in one and one-quarter, five or ten grains. Do NOT use if sensitive to aspirin; use Tylenol.

2. If the area is itchy and red, give an antihistamine (see pp. 207–208 and 275).

3. If the area is very swollen or hot, apply ice (not heat).

4. If the area is painful, red, itchy and swollen, do all of the above. A sling also might help if the arm is very painful.

Be very certain to tell your physician the exact extent and duration of the reaction *before* the next injection of allergy extract is given.

For a mild or severe reaction to traditional allergy-extract therapy affecting any body area other than the site of the injection, do the following:

1. If you are still in the physician's office, *immediately* ask his nurse or secretary if your child can be seen again by the doctor.

2. If you are on your way home, *immediately* stop the car and give your child an antihistamine *and* an asthma medicine, if you have both. Try *always* to carry these medicines in your car. Return to your physician's office.

3. If you are already home, give your child his usual antihistamine or asthma medicine *first,* then call the physician who gave the injection.

4. If, for some reason, you are very alarmed, in addition to the

---

[1] As mentioned previously, local itching at the exact area of the treatment is not abnormal.

previous suggestion also place a tourniquet above the site of the injection and apply ice. Immediately take your child to the nearest physician or hospital. Release the tourniquet for a few seconds every ten minutes until medical help is obtained.

Please be assured that severe reactions to extract-injection treatments seldom occur, but if they do, it is certainly better to know what to do to help your child immediately.

**Why would a severe abnormal reaction to an allergy injection occur?**

This could occur if the extract medicine happened to be injected into an area *near* a blood vessel. The physician or nurse always pulls back on the syringe before injecting to be certain that it is not being given intravenously, but sometimes it is not possible to know how close the nearest blood vessel is. If the extract is injected near a large blood vessel, it would have the same effect as suddenly being exposed to a very large amount of the substances which cause allergies, and the result is the abrupt occurrence of allergic symptoms. This is called an "allergic reaction" to an extract treatment.

**How often do severe, abnormal, allergic reactions occur from traditional extract treatment?**

Very rarely, because the dosage is gradually increased at regular intervals and is initially adjusted by the allergist.

**How can you help to prevent your child from having a reaction to an allergy treatment?**

Watch your child while you are waiting in the doctor's office after a traditional treatment has been given. Notify your physician if any *sudden* allergic symptoms occur. Watch your child's arm that evening and possibly the next day after the treatment. If there is unusual swelling or redness, be certain to tell the physician about it *before* the next treatment is given. If there was an extreme reaction to any treatment, call the doctor and discuss it. Such a reaction may alter the date for the next treatment.

If a bioassay titration end-point treatment causes symptoms, they are usually mild and occur most often within ten minutes. Stop further therapy until your doctor is notified.

**What reactions are not caused by allergy-extract treatments?**

Fever is almost never caused by an extract. If one is noted shortly after a treatment, it usually indicates a coincidental infection. Allergic symptoms which start to occur more than two hours after the treatment are usually not related to it. It would be most rare for a child to wheeze only on the day *after* an injection treatment. However, if these types of reactions are noted, they should be discussed with the allergist.

**Should any precautions be taken when a child receives any type of allergy treatment?**

Yes. Although reactions to allergy-extract treatments seldom occur, to be forewarned is to be forearmed. Do the following and don't worry.

1. Always wait 20 minutes in the physician's office after the actual time of the extract treatment. Wait even if the treatments have been received for years and no difficulty has ever been noted. If the office is too crowded, wait outside, possibly in your car. If a severe "abnormal" reaction occurs, it is most apt to start within 20 minutes and your physician knows exactly what to do and can readily give the necessary medicine *if you are still in the office*. Many parents do not wait because they live only five minutes away from the doctor's office. This is foolish since they may not find the physician in the office by the time they return.

2. When a child is being treated, an adult should always be with him. The child should also be watched for about two hours[1] after the treatment is given, because an occasional late reaction occurs. Strenuous exercise should be avoided for at least two hours after the injection. Try to make the allergy-treatment appointments on days when there is no football practice or swimming.

3. Always carry antihistamines (a medicine for nose, eye or skin allergy) and an asthma medicine in the car or your purse so that, if sudden allergic symptoms develop while in the car or on the way home, both medicines can immediately be given. (See pp. 207–212 and 275.) If a reaction occurs, it might start with a simple sneeze or nose rub but often wheezing and coughing follow in a few minutes. The reverse can also occur. This can happen even if the child has never had asthma before.

4. Try Alka-Seltzer Antacid Formula without aspirin.

**What mild symptoms may occasionally occur after a *traditional* allergy-extract treatment?**

Some parents repeatedly note that their children's appetites are diminished or that they are tired, listless or have a headache for several hours after an injection. This is often eliminated by lowering the dosage of the extract.

---

[1] Allpyral extracts can cause reactions several hours after the treatment.

## Does a child's reaction to a traditional extract ever change?

Yes. As time passes most patients become more and more tolerant of the extract and have less and less of a local reaction in the injection area. In rare instances, the reverse occurs and the same dosage of extract that a child has received for years suddenly appears to be too strong. If this occurs, check with your allergist.

## Should a patient receive a traditional allergy treatment if he has a slight infection (such as a cold or sore throat)?

Yes. When someone has a history of wheezing with each infection, the injection treatment is more necessary than at other times, for this is when the child is most apt to wheeze. The allergy treatment should not be given when a child is in a toxic condition (very ill or with a high fever). Once the illness is no longer acute, treatment should be given. Some young children who have asthma wheeze so often that if a physician waited until the chest was clear before treating such a child, treatment would seldom be given. In any particular patient, however, the final decison must be that of your physician.

## If a child is wheezing slightly, can he receive an allergy-extract treatment?

Yes. However, if the wheeze is severe, the asthma should be treated and no extract given. Let the physician in charge decide.

## How many years must children receive traditional allergy treatment?

This varies greatly with individual children and the severity of their disease. In general, treatments will be required for a longer period if the symptoms started early in life, if there were many manifestations of allergies and if the child was severely ill with these. However, if the problem is mild and seasonal (for example, from the middle of August to late September), only three years of treatment may be required. Treatments are generally discontinued when a child has had no symptoms *from exposure to substances for which he has been treated* for a full two or three years. Some children require treatments most of their lives. Keep records, as suggested on pages 24–25, to help your allergist decide when to stop treatments.

With *bioassay titration* therapy, some patients appear to be able to stop therapy relatively soon, sometimes within one to three years.

**What happens if a child's treatments are discontinued before the physician recommends it?**

If the child is fortunate, symptoms may not recur. In many patients who stop treatments too soon, the previously noted problems recur within several months. In most of these patients resumption of previous treatment causes the former improvement to be noted again.

**If a child is wheezing or having mild nasal symptoms prior to a traditional allergy treatment, how can his parents tell if a reaction to the injections is occurring?**

The wheezing or nasal symptoms would become much worse, usually within two hours of the time after the injection was received. The area of the injection treatment is frequently very red and swollen if a patient has a reaction to an extract-injection treatment.

**Do patients sometimes need their traditional extract treatments more often than every four weeks after they are receiving a maintenance dosage of extract?**

Yes. While most children do well on a four-week treatment schedule, some patients seem to *need* their treatments more often. A parent will note that repeatedly, a few days or a week or two before the next treatment is due, allergy symptoms recur and medicine is needed. This might indicate that the treatments need to be given more often. If the symptoms frequently occur three days before the monthly injection is due, the child should be receiving the injection treatments every 25 days, not every 28 days. In a few months, a 28-day schedule may be tried again and, if no symptoms are noted between injections, the child can continue receiving treatments every four weeks.

With *titration end-point* therapy, after the initial response, the treatment is given as often as necessary, usually on a daily or weekly basis.

**Why might a physician suddenly change a child from a monthly to a weekly schedule for extract treatments?**

The most common reason would be an attempt to raise the extract-dosage level in order to give the child more protection, for example, during a pollinating season. If a child is receiving the maximum amount of extract and continues to have symptoms at a certain time of the year, more frequent treatments at the troublesome period sometimes relieve symptoms. As soon as the season which causes symptoms has passed, the interval between the injections can again be increased to three or four weeks or whatever your allergist recommends.

**Why should the dosage of traditional extract be decreased and then increased again when new, fresh extract is started?**

Fresh extract is usually stronger than the extract which has been used for one or one and one-half years. Even though extracts are kept refrigerated, deterioration is only delayed, not prevented. There are also pollen differences each year. Just as a grape crop may make better wine in one year than in another, the ragweed extract made from one year's crop may be more or less allergenic than in previous years. An extract mixture is generally made with the same amount of the same ingredients each year, but because each component varies slightly, several extra visits for "build-up" injections are required with each new supply of extract. Usually, extracts expire in one or at most one and one-half years after preparation and *must* be replaced at that time.

**Can a mother or friend who is a nurse give a child his allergy-injection treatments?**

There is no unanimity of opinion. Some physicians in some countries allow patients to give their own treatments. Most allergists prefer that doctors give traditional allergy injections because, if a reaction occurs, a cool head, experience and emergency equipment must be readily available. Savings in time and money cannot compare with the anxiety caused by a severe reaction. The newer, controversial titration end-point treatment rarely causes problems and patients routinely treat themselves with drops under the tongue or arm/leg injections.

**What can you do if traditional pollen therapy does not seem to help?**

Try to investigate other forms of treatment.

The judicious use of drugs may resolve the problem. The newer titration therapy may give such relief that drugs are unnecessary or less essential. Be sure the bedroom is allergy-free. Also wash pollen from hair at bedtime.

**Should your child receive traditional allergy-injection treatments from your pediatrician or the allergist?**

This is not easy to answer. Some pediatricians or allergists prefer to administer treatments personally to all their patients. Some ask parents to decide, because one physician may be closer to the child's home or less expensive. For the average patient, it does not matter who gives the actual extract treatments *provided* that a physician is present when they are given. If a particular child has any difficulty when receiving injection treatments, these should definitely be given by the allergist acquainted with his case, at least until the problem is solved. Allergists who personally give extract treatments are in a better position to provide regular supervision of all aspects related to a child's allergies. If your child is not entirely well, do not hesitate to ask the doctor to examine him *before* the extract is given.

### Can two different extracts be mixed in the same syringe?

Yes. At times they can, if both extracts are similar. Most, but not all, allergists prefer to mix several allergenic substances in the same syringe.

### What is a bacterial vaccine?

This is a medicine which is composed of killed or weakened bacteria (germs). It is often prescribed for children who have frequent colds associated with their asthmatic episodes. This medicine can be combined with other allergenic substances in a treatment extract or can be injected separately. There are two major types available. One is a stock vaccine which is often composed of many types of killed bacteria which commonly cause infections. The other is called an autogenous bacterial vaccine and is made from the germs found in a child's own lung mucus or secretions. This mucus for vaccine preparation is often obtained during bronchoscopy, a hospital procedure which allows the physician to look directly into a child's lungs. The effectiveness of these vaccines is continually being challenged but there seems to be little doubt that some children do stop having infections after they have been used. They are currently used infrequently, not because they are unsafe but because their effectiveness is still questionable.

### What is a repository or long-acting extract treatment?

One type is a water-in-oil emulsion mixture of an allergy extract in a special oil solution so that it is absorbed more slowly after it has been injected. This type can cause undesirable side effects.

A second type[1] (Allpyral) uses alum to precipitate the allergenic substance before it is put in suspension. It provides a slower rate of absorption of the allergenic substances. Fewer injections of extract are needed to give the desired amount of protection.

The superiority of these more slowly absorbed extracts is not completely or clearly substantiated at the present time.

---

[1] Allpyral extracts can cause reactions several hours after the treatment.

**Does it harm an extract to be at room temperature?**

A *sterile* extract can be mailed within several days without cause for concern. However, extracts should be kept refrigerated whenever possible.

**Does it harm an extract to be frozen?**

It would be best if extracts were not frozen. Freezing can cause a clear extract to become cloudy. Allpyral extracts are normally cloudy and should not be frozen.

**Can a blood test tell how to treat a patient?**

Yes, sometimes. The RAST test (see p. 185) shows great promise in replacing the need for the traditional skin test for pollen, mold and dust types of allergy. Drs. Nalebuff and Fadal have developed a method to determine directly the "correct" treatment dose, similar to the *Bioassay Titration Method* using the RAST. This method may miss slight allergies and would not detect the more common, delayed type of food sensitivity. The shortcomings of these newer methods are now being evaluated. In time, it would appear that a blood test will help detect the major causes of an allergy, indicate the correct dosage for treatment and enable the patient to treat himself with injections, drops under the tongue or a nasal spray.

**Do symptoms ever recur after your allergist recommended stopping injection treatments?**

Yes. This, however, is the exception and not the rule. Many children remain symptom-free if they were really well for a full two to three years before stopping treatments. Occasionally symptoms recur in a year or more; new extract treatments will generally cause the symptoms to subside again.

# PART FIVE

# Commonly used medicines and their relation to allergy

CHAPTER 12 answers common questions about medicines in general. It tells how soon and how long medicines act and when they should be taken. The specific types of drugs used to treat various types of allergies are discussed. Included are descriptions of the usual desirable and undesirable effects these drugs have.

Chapter 13 is a section on immunization which will be of particular help to parents of allergic children. Problems in relation to an allergy to horse serum are covered in detail.

Chapter 14 explains which drugs often cause allergies, and what types of problems this kind of sensitivity can cause. Advice is given concerning the prevention of future exposure to potentially highly allergenic medicines.

# CHAPTER 12

# *Medicines used to treat allergies*

## MEDICINE IN GENERAL

**How can you tell when you should give your child a medicine?**

Have faith in your own judgment. If your child complains of a slight headache but is playing and acting normally, or if he coughs three times and not again, medicine is not needed. But if your child complains of symptoms for more than a few minutes and obviously is not acting like himself, give the appropriate medicine as recommended by your physician.

**How can you tell when to stop giving a medicine, once it has been started?**

This would depend upon which medicine was taken and why it was given. If a headache is gone, stop giving aspirin. If the nose is fine after one antihistamine tablet, don't give more. At times, your physician will advise you to use medicine for several days; this should be given *exactly* as recommended. Parents frequently tend to use a sample of antibiotic medicine (such as penicillin) and do not fill the prescription for more medicine as recommended because the child seems better. This is a serious mistake. If antibiotics are not taken for an adequate period of time, the same infection is very apt to recur. This particular infection may then be more difficult to treat. (A relapse sometimes occurs after adequate antibiotic therapy, however, and may be caused by a different organism not sensitive to the first antibiotic. Fungal infections, for example, are often a problem after antibiotics are given.)

The germs causing most infections are mainly bacteria, viruses or fungi.

**What is the difference between a "four-times-a-day" medicine and one to be given every six hours?**

By "four-times-a-day" your physician generally means that the drug should be given at 8:00 A.M., noon, 4:00 P.M., and 8:00 P.M. If your child arises at 7:00 A.M., give each dose of medicine one hour earlier. Try to divide the hours your child is awake into four equal parts and give the medicines at these intervals. If the physician recommends that medicines be given every six hours, this usually means exactly that. Start at 8:00 A.M., repeat at 2:00 P.M. and at 8:00 P.M., with the next dose due at 2:00 A.M. If you feel your child is not so ill that you want to interrupt his sleep, check with your doctor about omitting the 2:00 A.M. dose.

**When should medicines be given during the night?**

For the most part, this is required only if your child is extremely ill. If he has a severe infection, it is often necessary for him to take the antibiotic every few hours, including a dose during the night, so that there is a constant high blood level of that drug. This is especially essential in the early treatment of an infection.

Asthmatic children who are *sleeping quietly* should not be awakened at night to give them medicine to control their wheezing. Disturbing their sleep is often the cause of immediate asthma and coughing. One major disadvantage of many theophylline drugs for asthma is that they help for only about six hours. Newer forms with longer-lasting benefits are just beginning to be used.

**How long does it take for a medicine to have its effect?**

Most allergy medicines taken by mouth act in about 20 minutes. Some will be slightly quicker or slower (up to 30 minutes or so). Liquids work faster than pills. Rectal suppositories are quite variable in their rate of absorption and may start to help in 20 minutes or several hours.

Some oral sprays used to treat asthma act immediately but the duration of activity is short, perhaps varying from 20 minutes to about two hours, depending on the type used.

**What is the duration of a medicine's action?**

This varies, but if the medicine is to be taken every four hours, it should last about four hours. A medicine to be taken every eight to twelve hours should maintain its effect for at least eight and possibly for twelve hours. Long-acting medicines, in particular, may not always give relief for as long as they should. If an eight-to-twelve-hour medicine seems to help for only four hours, check with your physician.

**What do you do if a medicine does not relieve the symptoms for which it was taken?**

Contact your physician. Maybe it has not been used long enough, or a different medicine might be needed.

**How can you decide which of several sample medicines help?**

Give one to your child and see if the symptom for which it was given lessens in about half an hour. Several antihistamines may have to be tried before an effective one is found. When your child has nasal symptoms, try the first and if there is no improvement after four or six hours you can try another. Do not give more than one antihistamine at exactly the same time. This would be comparable to taking several brands of aspirin at the same time and could cause an overdose. If questions arise, check with your doctor.

**What do you do if the medicine lessens the symptoms for which it was taken but causes some other undesirable effect?**

If the medicine helps but creates an unpleasant side effect, check with your physician. Some of these side effects are at times beneficial. If an antihistamine makes a child very sleepy, it should certainly not be used during the day, but this would be a fine medicine to use at bedtime. If the medicine does not help your child's symptoms and has an undesirable side effect, discontinue using it and contact your physician.

**What unsuspected additives in medicines can cause allergies?**

Colors or dyes at times cause allergies. Some children, for example, have allergic symptoms if they eat or drink anything that is red or yellow, including not only medicines but also foods or drinks. The color of some dyed pills can be rinsed off with water. Corn or sugar in drugs can cause symptoms in some children. Some children are allergic also to flavors like licorice, root beer, cherry, cinnamon or orange.

**Can several medicines be taken at the very same time?**

Yes, if they are given for entirely different reasons and do not contain the same substances, *usually* it would be safe. For example, if a child wheezes, has a stuffy nose, a fever and a sore throat, he can simultaneously be given asthma medicine for his wheezing, an antihistamine, aspirin and an antibiotic (for the infection). If there is ever any question check with your physician. It is possible for nasal, cough and asthma medicine each to contain one drug in common and, therefore, be certain to check with your physician before the medicines are used together for the first time. Occasionally two entirely unrelated drugs have some unusual effect in the body if they are taken together, but this can be avoided by asking your doctor's advice.

### What are suppositories?

These are medicines to be given rectally. They are frequently used when children cannot take medicine by mouth because of vomiting. Be sure to remove the aluminum-foil outer wrapping and grease them with Vaseline or cold cream before inserting. They may feel greasy, but they hurt if they are given without extra lubrication. Finger cots are inexpensive covers for the finger used to insert the suppository. These can be obtained at any pharmacy. Soft suppositories are impossible to insert. If this is a problem, rub the suppository on an ice cube or put it into the freezer for a few minutes. The insertion of a suppository can cause a feeling similar to the need for moving one's bowels. To prevent this, push the suppository in as far as you can and then give it a little flip sideways. This doesn't hurt any more than taking a temperature rectally or having a bowel movement. If the child immediately wants to move his bowels, try to have him rest on his side for a few minutes. If you insert a suppository and your child moves his bowels in a few minutes, check with your doctor to find out when the next one should be given. Suppositories can frequently be inserted into a sleeping child without waking him.

Suppositories are given for various unrelated medical problems. One type is often prescribed for a child who is vomiting. Some antibiotics are now available in rectal form for children who are vomiting.

### How important is it to give medicine at intervals recommended by the doctor?

In many cases it is crucial to give medicine every four or six hours, or exactly as your physician suggested. Antibiotics, for example, usually are most effective if they are taken at regular intervals, so that blood level remains high enough to kill the germs or prevent their multiplying. As a medicine is absorbed into the bloodstream, it gradually rises to a peak and then starts to fall. If medicines are taken properly, the blood level of the drug would not be allowed to fall below the effective level. If the level does fall too low, germs causing the infection again can have a harmful effect.

If asthma medicines are not taken as recommended, the air tubes can continually go into and out of spasm and you will see little improvement in your child.

## Are there many children who cannot take aspirin?

No, most children are not allergic to aspirin; it usually occurs more frequently in adults. It is sometimes difficult for parents or physicians to tell whether a child's wheeze is from aspirin or the infection. Adults who cannot tolerate aspirin often have wheezing, nasal polyps (swellings of wet tissue inside the nose) and a sensitivity to yellow-dyed food substances. Patients who cannot take aspirin (acetylsalicylic acid) should use an aminophenol drug or aspirin substitutes such as Apomide, Tylenol or Tempra. This is available as a liquid or in tablet form without a prescription.

## How important is it to take a medicine at the times directed?

If the prescription specifies when medicine is to be taken, every effort should be made to follow the instructions exactly. Usually the reason for specific directions is that the drug is most effective if taken as recommended. If you take it at some other time it may not be absorbed as well, or could possibly cause abdominal discomfort. Some medicines help most if given immediately before, after or between meals. With others, this is unimportant.

## Do all drugstores charge the same for medicines?

No. You can shop for drugs just as you shop for foods or even physicians. If you buy a specific brand of medicine, there cannot be a substitute and the prices can or should be comparable regardless of where you buy it. If, however, you buy a medicine such as penicillin and the brand is not specified, the price could vary greatly from one drugstore to another. Some might give you a product which costs more because it is well advertised or because it is truly a better product. They might sell you an inexpensive brand that is less costly because the manufacturer is not well known, or perhaps the product itself may be inferior in some way.

The best example would be aspirin. You can buy this item at many prices. The inexpensive kind contains the same medicine (acetylsalicylic acid) as the expensive. The inexpensive tablets, however, might crumble after six months and the expensive ones might have an antacid added so that you will not have abdominal discomfort after taking the preparation. As with most purchases, you get what you pay for and quality costs more. Most physicians will prescribe brands of medicines if they feel it is important.

**When should a child switch from liquid to tablet medicine?**

This depends upon the child. If the liquid has a pleasant taste, there is no necessity for change. If the liquid has a disagreeable flavor, and a child cannot swallow a tablet, there may be some chewable forms of the medicine available. If a child *can* swallow a tablet, this or a tasteless capsule is usually preferred. If a child will not or cannot take any pill form of medicine and the liquid has a bad taste, try putting the liquid into a quarter of a glass of a strongly flavored fruit juice such as grape or prune.

**How can you teach a child to swallow a pill?**

Most children who are about seven years old can learn to take pills. Tell the child that pills have very little taste in comparison with many liquid medicines and this will give him the incentive. Buy some small candy which is about pill size. Place one in the center of the tongue as far back as you can. Have the child take a large drink of water. The "pill" will often be easily washed over the back edge of the tongue. Drugstores now sell special cups containing a little pill compartment to help young children who have difficulty swallowing pills. The pill (or tablet) is placed in the compartment, the cup is filled with water or juice and the child consumes both simultaneously.

**How can a child take a capsule medicine that cannot be swallowed?**

Open the capsule and place its contents in some jam, peanut butter, a marshmallow, on ice cream or in a cream-filled chocolate candy. Try not to place it in a food which causes allergies in your child.

**Can you safely discard allergy medicine if your child has had no symptoms for a long time?**

Please don't. Children may have no allergic symptoms for months, but then suddenly have an asthma attack or a bout of hay fever. These episodes may occur at a most inconvenient time, as when drugstores are closed. Try never to be without all the medicines which your child may need for an emergency allergic episode. Always carry them on trips or vacations. Most allergy medicines in tablet or clear-liquid form retain their potency for long periods of time. If there is any doubt, check with your pharmacy or physician.

**If drugstore allergy medicine helps, why should your child see an allergist?**

If your child has mild symptoms and such medicine helps, your child doesn't need an allergist. Parents, however, sometimes cannot evaluate which problems are mild and which are severe. The solution to a child's allergic problem is not only to treat the symptoms, *but also eliminate what is causing them.* To do this, the help of an allergist is often necessary. Caution should be exercised so that the choice of your child's medicine is always that of your physician, not that of a relative, friend or druggist.

## ANTIHISTAMINES

### What are antihistamines?

This medicine helps to relieve nose, eye or ear symptoms of allergies and skin allergies which cause itching resulting from hives or eczema. (Antihistamines can also relieve the itching of mosquito or insect bites and chicken-pox lesions.) Antihistamines decrease tissue swelling and mucous production. For example, the same antihistamine could help either a stuffy nose (caused by tissue swelling) or a runny nose (caused by excessive mucus).

### Are non-prescription, drugstore antihistamines helpful?

Yes. Usually these are milder forms of what the physician would prescribe. If they help, and are used as directed, they should be safe. Examples are Chlortrimeton, chewable Novahistine or Tacaryl liquid, Ryna or Triaminic.

### Are antihistamines ineffective at times?

Yes. Antihistamines are all similar in their action but there are several different chemical types. If one does not help, a change to another which is quite different chemically may prove to be most effective.

When hay fever or eczema symptoms are very severe, no antihistamine may be helpful. Many different chemical types may be tried without success. After the child has received extract treatments, these same medicines may relieve less severe allergy symptoms completely.

### In which forms are antihistamines sold?

There are liquids which last from four to 12 hours, depending on the type. There are chewable pills which are most convenient for children of school age, because these can be carried by reliable children and taken without water when needed. They should be chewed for the best effect. Unlike tablets, capsules have no taste when swallowed and older children tend to prefer these.

**What bad effects do antihistamines have?**

The most frequent one is drowsiness or sleepiness. If this is noted, but it relieves the nose, eye or skin allergic symptoms, use the medicine at bedtime. During the daytime, try half the recommended dosage and it may be effective without causing drowsiness. If this does not help, check with your physician and another chemical type of antihistamine can be prescribed. At times, when an antihistamine is first taken, it causes sleepiness, but after a few days this no longer occurs. In rare cases, antihistamines might cause abdominal discomfort or a dry mouth.

Another common side effect is that antihistamines can alter one's coordination, so they should never be taken before a child engages in competitive sports. (Exercise will frequently clear the nose temporarily and this sometimes means that medication might not be needed.)

**Do antihistamines ever lose their effectiveness?**

Yes, sometimes if the same one is used three or four times a day for several months the symptoms may no longer be relieved. Contact the physician for another type of antihistamine. After a few months of not using the original antihistamine, your child may find that it is again effective.

**Can adults and children have a different reaction to the same antihistamine?**

Yes. Paradoxically, adults are sometimes more sensitive and seem to become sleepy with a child's dose, while a child occasionally can take an adult dose without becoming drowsy or having adverse symptoms.

**What happens if a child takes a marked excess of antihistamine?**

Usually he becomes very sleepy. If there is an extreme overdose, this drowsiness is replaced by excitation and restlessness. If a child should drink the medicine by error, first try to induce vomiting by putting your finger down his throat; then contact your physician or nearest hospital or call the Poison Control Center.

**Do antihistamines help asthma?**

Theoretically they should, but usually they are not ordered because they tend to dry mucus and it would be undesirable to thicken and dry the mucus in a child's lungs. They can safely be used to treat nasal symptoms which accompany asthma if the proper asthmatic medicine is given at the same time.

## NOSE DROPS

### Do nose drops or sprays help nasal or ear allergies?

Yes, they do. Antihistamines should be used first to see if they help your child's symptoms. Many physicians object to nose drops because they are often used excessively, causing nasal blockage. This is called "rhinitis medicamentosa." For this reason, they should be used only in selected instances when the nasal problem is severe. An example would be if a child could not sleep because of extreme nasal obstruction or stuffiness.

### How should nose drops be used?

They should be used no more often than three times a day for three days. (See p. 38 for exact details concerning how to use them.) After not using them for several days, they may again be given for three more days. This will prevent irritation of the inside of the nose. There are different strengths of Neo-Synephrine nose drops for infants, children and adults. No prescription is needed for Neo-Synephrine or Alconephrine. Afrin, Privine and Tyzine may be too strong for many children. Otrivin Pediatric Nose Drops are available by prescription and one application may be helpful for 12 or more hours.

## ASTHMA MEDICINES

### What types of asthma medicines are there?

Several. Most are given by mouth, in liquid, tablet or capsule form. Rectal suppositories are not recommended but liquid rectal medicines are sometimes necessary and effective. Aerosol-mist therapy is also available. This can be most helpful for young infants because it provides fast, easy relief of asthma. An example is the use of Bronkosol in a MaxiMyst machine.

### What do asthma medicines do?

They make breathing easier. They relax and enlarge the air tubes so that more air can pass in and out. They often make mucus thinner and easier to cough up. They also decrease the swelling of the lining of the air tubes, thus making it easier to breathe.

### What is Adrenalin (epinephrine)?

This is a medicine which is injected under the skin to relieve severe asthma. Most children feel better in a few seconds or minutes. There are some types whose effects last for only 20 minutes; others help immediately and are effective for as long as eight to 12 hours (for example, Asmolin or Susphrine). Any epinephrine preparation can increase a child's heartbeat but this is no more harmful than exercise. Many children are very pale and feel nervous after receiving epinephrine, but this is also normal.

### What is ephedrine?

This is the basic ingredient in most pills used to treat asthma. Its main effect is to enlarge the air tubes. If it causes excitement, lower the dosage by half or stop the drug and call your physician. Ephedrine causes nervousness, so this drug is mainly given in combination with a sedative such as phenobarbital. Ephedrine may occasionally cause insomnia or difficulty in urinating. If this is noted, discuss it with your physician.

Newer ephedrine-like drugs (*e.g.*, Bricanyl, Metaprel) supposedly have fewer side effects and a longer duration of action.

### Are there other drugs to use if your child cannot take ephedrine?

Yes. Orthoxine is a substitute, ephedrine-like drug.

### What is Aminophylline (theophylline)?

This is a medicine used in an oral liquid or pill form or as a suppository to help asthmatics breathe easier. Since the absorption of suppositories is unreliable, this form of medication is no longer recommended. Many liquid forms contain alcohol and have a rather unpleasant taste. If too much is taken, it can cause nausea and vomiting of a coffee-colored material, or extreme restlessness or agitation. If any of these symptoms occur, call your doctor. The medicine is sometimes administered intravenously to help control a severe asthmatic episode.

Surprisingly, Aminophylline preparations are currently popular in spite of the fact that the dose must be repeated every six hours and cannot be easily calculated. Blood or saliva theophylline levels must be monitored to be certain that patients are receiving the correct dosage of this drug.

### Are asthma mouth-spray aerosols effective?

Yes, but there is a tendency for older children to overuse them. They help in seconds and are liked for this reason, but their effect usually lasts for only a short while. This is why asthma pills which help for hours are preferable.

To use a mouth aerosol requires a degree of cooperation and coordination which most younger children, try as they may, simply do not have. For the spray to be effective, the lips must be tightly closed around the mouthpiece. The child must breathe through his nose and, as the air is passing into the lungs, the aerosol is released into the mouth so that it can also enter the lungs. The breath must then be held as long as possible, so that the medicine remains in the lungs. If the child immediately breathes out, the medicine will not have had enough time to help. If your child uses the spray and when he opens his mouth a cloud of white comes out, the medicine never reached the lungs and was ineffective.

If sprays are used too often (usually more than three or four times a day) they are seldom helpful; also, they can irritate the throat, cause an upset stomach or headache and *actually make asthma worse in some patients*. For these reasons many physicians do not recommend them. Sprays are best saved only for emergencies, if they must be used at all. If they don't help, contact your physician.

Aerosol-mist solutions administered by a MaxiMyst machine (available at drugstores) are very helpful for infants or children who refuse medicines. Bronkosol and water make a spray which may help as quickly as Adrenalin by injection. This combination requires little patient cooperation.

### What is the difference between a cough medicine and an asthma medicine?

Many cough medicines are mixtures containing any combination of the following: (1) a mucus-thinning medicine; (2) a mucus-drying agent; (3) a cough suppressant; and (4) a tissue-shrinking medicine. Asthma medicines are also mixtures of several drugs which make breathing easier. Both cough and asthma medicines at times can contain some of the same drugs. Therefore, you must check with your doctor, if necessary, to be certain that these two drugs can be given at the same time.

### Should asthmatics use morphine, codeine or similar drugs?

Not usually. At times these can interfere with normal breathing and make asthma or an allergic cough worse. Codeine is prescribed mainly when it is desirable to stop a nightly, dry, irritating cough associated with an infection.

### What is Intal (cromolyn sodium)?

This drug was also previously marketed under the name of Aarane. It is a new, safe, white powder which is deeply inhaled into the lungs.

It often helps asthma caused by dust, pollen and molds, and sometimes aids patients with intrinsic asthma of unknown origin. In Canada and Europe, it is also used to treat eye, nose and food allergy.

Intal is the *before* drug. It *prevents* asthma if it is given a few minutes *before* exercise, emotional upsets or exposure to pets, allergenic foods, cold air, dusty places or Christmas trees. It will not immediately help a patient who is already wheezing. It must be used several times a day for several days before it will help asthma that has already occurred. It should be used *before* and *during* vacations and pollen seasons. In this manner, asthma sometimes can be prevented.

Intal is safe to use with other drugs which relieve asthma. It is sometimes beneficial because it decreases or eliminates the need for cortisone. Its safety during pregnancy is not known. Side effects of the drug are noted in 25 per cent of patients. These can include headache, hives, abdominal pain, diarrhea, vomiting, insomnia, depression and a runny nose. If these symptoms occur, consult your physician.


## STEROIDS OR CORTISONE DRUGS

**What is cortisone (a steroid)?**

This is a most powerful medicine used to treat allergies and many other diseases. It sometimes is the critical drug used to save lives. Like many strong drugs, it has great potential for helping a child, but it can also be very harmful. This drug should never be taken unless it is given *under a physician's close supervision*. Its major function is to diminish inflammation by decreasing swelling and redness which can occur in almost any area of the body for multiple reasons. This drug relieves but certainly does not cure allergy.

**When is cortisone prescribed?**

It is used mainly when a child cannot engage in normal activities of everyday living in spite of his using common medicines for allergies. It is essential in the treatment of some life-threatening or distressing allergic emergencies.

**Are cortisone skin medications dangerous?**

Generally not. They are most frequently used in low concentrations on relatively small areas of skin, with a mainly local effect.

**Is there a difference in cortisones?**

Yes, there is a great variation in the potency or strength of various cortisone salves or tablets. Only your physician can decide which your child needs and for how long a time.

### How much danger is there if cortisone is taken in large doses but for only a few days?

Usually very little. In an emergency situation, the drug is often administered this way; as soon as the child is better, the dose is quickly reduced and, if possible, stopped.

### Is stopping a cortisone drug ever a problem?

Yes. It is often very difficult to discontinue using this medicine, especially if the drug has been used for weeks or months. Each time the dosage is lowered, the child's symptoms, such as asthma or eczema, become worse. This is a real challenge for a physician and is a major reason why many physicians are most reluctant to start a child on this drug. *Never* suddenly stop any cortisone drug, except ointment, unless your physician has specifically advised you to do so. Under certain circumstances the drug *must* be tapered off and stopped very gradually.

### What undesirable minor effects can cortisone have?

It can cause acne, hairiness of the face or body, increased appetite, weight gain, abdominal pain and a rise in blood pressure, cataracts, dry mouth, fatigue, leg cramps and increased perspiration. Sometimes the breasts or anus will itch, bloating is noted, the face becomes round, or there is a hump on the back of the neck. Sometimes there will be sugar in the urine temporarily. There may be insomina. Growth in height is decreased. These problems usually disappear if the cortisone is stopped, or if the dosage is lowered sufficiently.

### What is one of the most serious problems which cortisone causes?

It tends to allow infections which normally would be confined to a certain body area to spread to other parts of the body. In addition, it gives a child a feeling of well-being. This combination is possibly dangerous, since it means an infection can spread and the parents may not have any warning, because the child feels fine. For this reason, again, children on cortisone should be closely and regularly supervised by their physician *regardless* of how well they feel. If a child is taking this drug and feels unwell in any way or develops a fever, contact your physician.

### Can cortisone affect the growth of a child?

Yes. In large doses, for prolonged periods of time, the growth in height can be less than normal when using certain cortisone drugs.

When the drug is stopped, however, there will generally be a sudden, rather fast, compensatory growth spurt in height, provided that the child is still at the age when his bones are growing. This tendency to interfere with growth in height can be diminished if the dosage of the drug is very low or if certain cortisone drugs are given every other day rather than daily. Some children are so ill that the physician has a very difficult decision to make. In spite of its effect on growth and other problems connected with this drug, cortisone is sometimes essential so that a child can live a relatively normal life.

### What about the inhaled cortisone powder, Vanceril?

This new drug can be breathed into the lungs to help control asthma. The absorption of the drug is less, and therefore the side effects are diminished. When patients improve, the allergist's aim is to try to convert the patient from oral cortisone to this inhaled cortisone. If a patient feels unwell during this adjustment, his physician should be contacted. The major side effect of the drug is thrush, or white patches on the inside of the mouth, which often can be prevented by rinsing the mouth after the drug is used.

### What is the danger of having chicken pox when a child is on cortisone therapy?

As mentioned before, infections tend not to stay localized when a patient is on cortisone, so chicken pox, which usually appears on the skin, can also possibly occur inside the body and make a child very ill. For this reason, it is always safer for a child to use this drug only after he has already had this childhood illness. While chicken pox may present no problem, measles (in a patient taking steroids) may prove a challenge and cause serious medical problems.

### How long can a child remain on cortisone therapy?

Some children are on cortisone for many years and into adulthood. This is certainly not desirable but is absolutely essential in severely ill patients.

### Is it ever necessary to resume cortisone after it has been discontinued?

Yes. The most common reason is that a child develops another extremely severe allergic episode, such as asthma, and the drug is necessary to help relieve and control the child's symptoms.

There are other occasions when this drug must be started again even though your child might not have a severe allergic problem. Let us suppose that your child was very ill with allergies or some other medical problem, and had to have this drug. If received in large amounts over a long period of time, it is possible that the adrenal glands, which make cortisone, would be affected. These glands can shrink and become smaller whenever a person receives cortisone medicine by mouth or injection. Normally, when the human body is under stress (such as when an operation is needed or there is a death in the family), these glands produce extra cortisone to help cope with the emergency need. If these glands, however, are not able to function adequately and produce the additional cortisone when it is needed, it must be supplied by your physician. For this reason, if your child has received this drug within the past six to 12 months and a serious emotional or medical situation arises, you should discuss it with *all* physicians caring for your child. Depending upon which cortisone drug your child took and for how long, your physicians will decide if more is necessary, and advise you accordingly.

**What are the names of some common cortisone preparations?**

betamethasone (Celestone)

dexamethasone (Decadron, Hexadrol, Gammacorten)

fludrocortisone (Florinef)

methylprednisolone (Medrol)

paramethasone (Haldrone)

prednisolone (Delta-Cortef, Predne-Dome)

prednisone (Deltasone, Delta-Dome)

triamcinolone (Aristocort, Kenacort)

cortisones combined with antihistamines are Aristomin, Dronactin and Metreton.

beclomethasone (Vanceril) aerosol

## MEDICINES FOR THE SKIN

**What relieves itching?**

Calamine decreases itching. This can be purchased without a prescription and can be applied locally on the skin as often as necessary. It should help hives, eczema, skin-test or allergy-extract treatment areas, chicken pox, mosquito or insect bites. Antihistamine tablets are also beneficial. Certain ointments contain substances such as tars to decrease itching. Also, try a paste of meat tenderizer for itchy insect bites.

### Does cortisone salve help eczema?

Yes. Most cortisone skin medications help decrease the itch *temporarily*. Customarily, they are used four to five times a day and should be applied *sparingly*. Place a little on the tip of your finger, dot in tiny specks about one-half inch apart over the affected area. Blend the specks together. A thin layer applied often is much better than a thick dab once a day.

### Do bath oils help dry skin?

Yes, to a degree, but most of the oil will remain in the tub (beware of slippery tubs!) or on the towel unless oils are applied after bathing and drying. The basic problem is not the outside of the skin but inside, and oils applied to the surface only help temporarily.

### Will skin medication prevent eczema from recurring?

No. Cortisone salves will only help the *present* rash to disappear. Whenever the rash reappears, the salve is re-applied. Eczema will continue appearing *until the cause of the rash is eliminated*. The cause, unfortunately, is often not determined. A food, yeast, mold or chemical sensitivity are common, unsuspected causes.

## ANTIBIOTICS

### Are there different kinds of antibiotics?

Yes. There are some which help defend the body against what is called gram-positive bacteria and another type which relieves those infections caused by gram-negative organisms. We have no antibiotic to use for common viral infections. When an infection is not helped by an antibiotic, it may not be that the wrong one was used but that no effective one is available. The only way to be somewhat certain about which antibiotic to use is to culture the infected area. This is costly and may take several days or longer, so that many infections are cultured only if they seem to persist and are difficult to treat.

### After starting an antibiotic, how long does it take before a child improves?

At times a child will be better in a few hours, although it often requires one or two days. If your child does not improve, always check again with your physician.

**Is there any danger in giving an antibiotic without having your child examined by a physician?**

Yes. Usually there would be no problem. However, let us assume, for example, that your child was wheezing and had pneumonia. If you started asthma medicine and an antibiotic, you could not tell, unless your child had been examined or unless an X-ray were taken, that your child had pneumonia. If this disease is only partially treated with an antibiotic, chest problems might linger for an extended period of time. After partial treatment, it might be very difficult to diagnose the true cause of the original infection and the reason for the child's prolonged illness.

**Is there any harm in giving an antibiotic for just one or two days whenever you feel that your child has an infection?**

Yes. Assuming the antibiotic is the correct one, it will kill or stop the growth of the bacteria or organisms causing the infection. In the first day or two, the most sensitive germs would be affected. The organisms least sensitive to an antibiotic will not be altered. If you stop an antibiotic after only two days, the stubborn or strong bacteria will be the major ones left, they will begin to multiply and in a few days the infection may recur. At that time the antibiotic used before may be very ineffective since the organisms causing the infection are now relatively resistant to this particular drug.

## DYE-COLORED MEDICINES

**Do the dyes in medicines cause illness?**

If parents notice that medicines which contain certain food colors (red, green, etc.) appear repeatedly to cause hyperactivity, irritability or other symptoms, the problem can be due to food coloring. The dye coating of some tablets can be removed by rinsing with water. Artificial flavors, sugars, corn or the drug contained in the liquid, pill or capsule also may be at fault. If you notice this type of problem, try Alka-Seltzer, *in gold foil* (without aspirin), and ask your physician for white or colorless medications. Crush tablets and place them in mashed potatoes or jelly for younger children.

**Are vitamins helpful for infection?**

The controversy rages on. Most allergists believe that vitamins are not helpful for infection. Lendon Smith recommends high doses of Vitamin C for viral infections which cannot be helped by antibiotics. If the dose is too high, diarrhea may occur. Merely stop the Vitamin

C if this happens and, when the diarrhea has subsided, resume the Vitamin C at a smaller dose. Smith suggests 100 mg. up to eight months, 200 mg. up to five years and 500 to 1,000 mg. over the age of five. Use this dose every two hours during waking hours for the first few days of an infection. See if it helps. Some physicians believe that allergies can be relieved by the use of Vitamin A and high doses of Vitamin C and the B vitamins, especially $B_6$ and pantothenic acid. More scientific studies are needed to properly evaluate the exact role of each vitamin for persons who tend to have allergies.

# CHAPTER 13

# *Immunizations*

**Which immunizations cause *no* special problems in allergic children?**

Pertussis (whooping cough), measles, diphtheria, plague (cholera) vaccine and polio (oral immunization). On rare occasions, severe reactions can be seen to any vaccine, in any patient. Although reactions to drugs occur more often in allergic children, immunizations are usually well tolerated.

**Which immunizations could cause special problems in allergic children?**

*1. Smallpox vaccination.*

Any child who has eczema or burns, impetigo or skin problems should not be vaccinated. There is, however, no need to vaccinate children at present.

*2. Vaccines.*

MEASLES, GERMAN MEASLES, MUMPS—These vaccines usually are grown on chick or duck tissue. Children who cannot eat eggs, chicken or duck or cannot come into contact with feathers or chicken without having an allergic reaction should not receive these vaccines. If they can eat eggs or chicken without difficulty, *even if* their allergy skin test was positive, the vaccine should be safe.

INFLUENZA—This vaccine is usually grown on egg or chick tissue. The United States Public Health Service recommends that this be received yearly by patients who have asthma or chronic lung disease. The vaccine is usually given some time between September and early December. Initially two injections are required but, subsequently, only one annual booster is needed.

TYPHUS—This vaccine is usually grown on egg media.

Children who cannot eat eggs or chicken or cannot come into contact with feathers or chicken without having allergic symptoms should not be given vaccine grown on chick or avian (bird or duck) tissue culture. Children who have obvious allergic problems related to contact with dogs or rabbits should not be given vaccines grown on the dog- or rabbit-kidney tissue cultures.

Children who have definitely been told that they are allergic to neomycin should avoid vaccines which contain this antibiotic.

If a child has a skin test revealing an allergy to eggs, chicken, rabbits, ducks, or feathers, but has *no obvious symptoms* when exposed to these substances, the vaccine is probably safe.

Recent preliminary research studies have indicated that children who develop symptoms from contact with eggs or dogs can safely be immunized with vaccines prepared on these media. At this time, however, immunization of such children cannot be routinely recommended and the advice of an allergist should be sought by parents who have any questions.

Measles vaccine should be avoided by children who are receiving steroids or by those children who have a generalized malignancy, such as leukemia.

### Does the routine immunization for tetanus (lockjaw) cause unusual problems in allergic children?

No. Any child can have a toxic reaction such as fever, swelling or malaise from an immunization. Most allergic children would not react differently than other children to tetanus toxoid. If the vaccine contained casein, a milk-sensitive patient might have symptoms.

If a toxic reaction occurs which seems to be unusually severe, a different brand of toxoid should be used the next time. Another help is to have your child receive his next immunization in divided doses. It might require a few more visits to the doctor before the prescribed amount is received, but the likelihood of a reaction would be diminished. Discuss it with your physician and let him make the necessary decision.

Some mixed diphtheria-tetanus (lockjaw) vaccines contain mercury and can cause symptoms in patients who have this type of sensitivity.

### What is the difference between tetanus toxoid and tetanus antitoxin?

Tetanus toxoid is a weakened, modified form of tetanus toxin, which is nontoxic and causes children to form protection against lockjaw. Tetanus antitoxin is animal serum which contains protection against lockjaw. This is given to children who will not have adequate time to prepare their own protection after possible exposure to tetanus from an injury or accident.

### When should children receive tetanus-toxoid immunizations?

Different schedules are used by physicians, but injections are often given at the following ages: two to three months, three to four months, four to five months, 15 to 18 months, and at three, six, and 12 years of age. All of these are usually given in conjunction with diphtheria-toxoid and pertussis vaccine except that the latter is omitted at six and 12 years.

If an injury occurs and a booster has been received within a year, an additional one is unnecessary. If more than one year has elapsed between the time of a booster and an injury, an additional booster would be indicated.

### What is horse serum?

This is part of the blood of horses. If you allow blood to coagulate, a red clot forms at the bottom and clear yellow serum rises to the top. The serum is the part of the blood which contains protection if a horse is immunized.

### Are some children allergic to horse serum?

Yes. This can be detected by testing in the skin or eyes. Any child allergic to horse serum should *always* wear a tag (see Appendix, p. 286) or carry a card stating that this is a problem.

### Why are some children allergic to horse serum?

We do not know but it could be related to the eating of meat. Children who are very allergic to many types of animals (*i.e.*, their fur or dander) are often allergic to horse serum.

### Which medical problems are treated with animal serum?

Snake and black widow spider bites, rabies, botulism, diphtheria, tetanus and gas gangrene are treated with antitoxins which can be made from various animals. Allergic children could have difficulty if they are sensitive to the animal type used to make one of these.

### How can the need for horse serum (to prevent lockjaw) be avoided if your child is allergic to it?

Merely be certain that your child receives tetanus-toxoid booster injections every ten years for the rest of his life. This would render the administration of tetanus antitoxin or horse serum unnecessary because your child could make protection against tetanus quickly if a booster toxoid injection were given at the time of an injury, such as stepping on a rusty nail or being hurt in an automobile accident.

**What happens if a child is given horse serum and is allergic to it?**

The child will probably develop a disease called serum sickness in about six to 21 days. This causes fever, swelling of the joints or body, an itchy rash and lymph-node swelling often necessitating hospitalization. Nervous system problems can occur, with weakness or pains in the arms or legs. If a child must receive horse serum, a sample of the blood can be studied to determine in advance whether serum sickness could develop. This is called a hemagglutination test, which only specially equipped laboratories can perform. Fatal reactions seldom occur from serum sickness, although some patients become extremely ill. (Tetanus, or lockjaw, can cause death.)

**Are there other animal sera which contain protection against tetanus?**

Yes, there is a cow, or bovine, type and also a human type, but these, too, can cause allergies. The human vaccine would cause less difficulty than those prepared from animals.

**Can an allergy-extract injection be given at the same time as an immunization?**

Yes, but if a reaction occurred it might be difficult to tell which was at fault. In general, an allergy injection might become red, swollen or painful but should not cause fever or a general feeling of malaise.

# CHAPTER 14

# *Allergies to drugs or medicines*

**Which drugs cause allergies?**

Any drug can cause an allergy. Some main offenders are:

aspirin
penicillin
sulfonamides or sulfa drugs
local anesthetics like the "caine" drugs, *e.g.*, procaine
iodides and bromides
antituberculous drugs
anticonvulsion drugs such as Dilantin, Tridione and Mesantoin
hormones such as ACTH or insulin
tranquilizers, especially phenothiazines
laxatives containing phenolphthalein
sedatives, such as barbiturates (phenobarbital)
any antibiotic
codeine, morphine

**What are typical allergic drug reactions?**

Hives, body swelling, nasal symptoms, asthma or skin rashes are typical. Certain drugs, such as some antibiotic tetracyclines, can cause photosensitivity. This means that slight exposure to sunlight causes a very severe sunburn. Hyperactivity and behavior problems appear to be related to food dyes, sugar and corn in drugs.

Drug reactions which occur infrequently would include drug fever, liver, kidney or blood changes.

**Can the allergist skin-test for drug allergies?**

Tests for some drugs can be done but these are not always reliable, although they can be useful, particularly in the case of penicillin. Some of the penicillin tests can be done in the child's skin and others can be done in the laboratory with blood samples. Skin testing is helpful in patients who have insulin, ACTH or liver-extract allergies.

Much research is being done in the field of drug-allergy detection at the present time. We cannot, however, accurately detect allergy to many drugs such as phenobarbital, most antibiotics, iodides or aspirin. In time this may be possible.[1]

### Are allergic children more likely to develop drug allergies?

There is some evidence that patients who have asthma may be more apt to develop aspirin or penicillin allergy, but, in general, there is no convincing proof that most types of drug reactions occur more frequently in allergic persons or families. Children have fewer allergies to such drugs as aspirin and penicillin than do adults.

Preliminary research indicates that *bioassay end-point titration* testing (Appendix V), with drugs to which patients are sensitive, may be helpful. The patient is treated with a dilution of the medicine to which he is sensitive. This sometimes relieves chronic symptoms when the drug cannot totally be avoided, *e.g.*, for the patient with chronic hives due to a penicillin allergy. Under some circumstances, this form of therapy appears to enable a patient to take a necessary drug in spite of a mild sensitivity to it.

### How soon after taking drugs do reactions occur and how long do these last?

Drug reactions can occur immediately or seven to 14 days after a drug is started and the reaction can at times last for months. In most patients, however, the reaction begins to subside several hours after the drug is discontinued. If a child is taking several medicines when a drug allergy develops, all of them may temporarily have to be stopped.

### What should your child do if he is allergic to a drug?

Two things should be done:

1. Avoid the drug in all forms and always double-check with the physician and the pharmacist to be certain the drug is not being received in an unrecognized form.

2. Have your child wear a medical name tag (see Appendix, p. 286) or, if your child is older, have him carry a card stating the name of the drug causing an allergy.

### Why does your child need to wear a medical name tag or carry a card regarding a drug allergy?

Because a child could have an accident and be unconscious upon

---

[1] Apparent drug reactions may not be due to the drug but to the dye, corn, sugar or flavoring in the medication. Newer testing methods help in detecting this type of problem.

arrival at a hospital where no one would know about his allergy. Younger children would normally be unable to state the name of the medicine to which they were allergic. A medical name tag can be obtained at most drugstores or through most medical supply houses.

### Are all drug reactions caused by allergy?

No. Some drugs irritate the bowel and cause diarrhea. This is a frequent undesirable side effect of many antibiotics, which is associated with the desirable major purpose of the drug, *i.e.,* to control or stop the infection.

Some drugs (aspirin, for example) cause nausea, dizziness and ringing in the ears if taken in very large doses. This could happen to anyone using this drug *in an excess dosage.* If a *very small amount* of this drug causes these reactions, the cause is not allergy but an intolerance. The child cannot "tolerate" a normal dose of this drug. True drug allergies cause symptoms which are in no way related to the normal response to the drug. If five grains of aspirin cause hives, this could be an allergy. If the same dose caused a child's ears to ring, it is an intolerance.

Some drugs provoke changes in the blood of certain children because of lack of a certain enzyme. This again is not an allergy but could be called an idiosyncrasy.

### What is the composition of aspirin?

It is acetylsalicylic acid. It is usually the acetyl portion of the drug which causes medical problems.

### Does aspirin cause allergy?

The exact mechanism of aspirin reactions is still controversial and for this reason a more correct term would be aspirin hypersensitivity, rather than allergy. Adults rather than children seem to be prone to a disease complex composed of asthma, nasal allergies, polyps and difficulty from some yellow dyes (used for orange- or yellow-colored foods, beverages and medicines).

Aspirin-sensitive patients should never try to use even the smallest amount of aspirin, because the results could be fatal.

### What are the symptoms of an aspirin hypersensitivity?

It has been known to cause nasal polyps, asthma, sinusitis, hives, body swelling, skin rashes, arthritis and blood problems in some persons.

## What do you give a child for a headache if he cannot use aspirin?

Give him an aspirin substitute. These are aminophenol-like drugs and your druggist can show you several types (Tylenol or Tempra), in both liquid and tablet form. No prescription is needed. Sodium salicylate is not harmful when used by most aspirin-sensitive patients.

## Do parents always know when their child reacts to aspirin?

No. It can be confusing because children tend to wheeze with infections. Thus, every time they begin to have an infection, they are given aspirin, and then they wheeze. A parent can wrongly assume that the infection is producing the wheeze when aspirin is the true cause. If your child takes aspirin and does not wheeze within three hours or have any medical problems, then there is probably no sensitivity to this drug. If you are in doubt, discuss it with your physician. Do not give your child aspirin if you think he cannot use it, because it could be dangerous. If a patient is sensitive to aspirin, merely placing a tablet on the tongue can be fatal.

## What should diabetic children do when they are allergic to insulin?

There are various types of insulin and your doctor will often try another type. Insulin preparations can be altered by heating so that they sometimes cause less allergy. Insulins are prepared from different animal species and if, for example, a child cannot use insulin from pigs (porcine), another type made from cows (bovine) might be satisfactory. (Similarly, ACTH derived from pigs cannot be used by some persons sensitive to pork products.)

Bioassay titration end-point testing sometimes enables patients to tolerate a form of insulin which causes symptoms.

## What problems do iodides sometimes cause?

Iodides are often given to wheezing children to help thin the chest mucus so that it can be coughed up more readily and easily. It can be part of a liquid or tablet mixture or could be in the form of a saturated solution of potassium iodide (SSKI). The latter can possibly stain a youngster's teeth, so brushing immediately after taking this medicine is recommended. The taste of iodide medicines is often quite disagreeable. For this reason it is best to give the medicine in a small quantity of liquid and then follow it with a pleasant-tasting beverage such as grape juice.

Some patients using this drug develop an acne-like rash or a swelling of their salivary or thyroid glands, hives, fever or other rashes. In many patients these problems subside when the medicine is stopped or the dosage is lowered.

Children with a sensitivity to iodides could possibly have problems when certain X-rays are made of their lungs (bronchograms), kidneys (intravenous pyelograms) or heart (angiocardiograms), because this drug is often used for outlining these organs. Unfortunately, we have no reliable, safe test for iodide sensitivity at the present time. In the future, bioassay titration end-point testing may prove helpful.

The mechanism causing iodide reactions is not well understood and there is evidence that such a sensitivity is not typically allergic in nature.

### Can local anesthetics cause allergy?

Yes, such drugs as procaine (novocain), Nupercaine or Benzocaine can cause reactions. This type of reaction is sometimes noted in children allergic to the sulfa variety of drugs. Lidocaine (xylocaine) is chemically different and often safe to use in these children for dental or other medical procedures when they cannot use the other "caine" preparations.

Preliminary evidence suggests that titration end-point testing with very weak solutions of a local anesthetic may be helpful. However, the testing requires hours, as gradually stronger dilutions are given every 15 minutes. If no problems arise during testing, the drug is probably safe.

### What are antibiotics?

These are medicines which help treat certain infections. Examples are penicillin, tetracyclines and erythromycins. One type of chemotherapeutic agent is a sulfonamide (sulfa). Antibiotics or chemotherapeutic drugs kill or hinder the growth of bacteria which cause infection. Different bacteria are sensitive to different antibiotics. Viral infections (for example, colds) are not helped by antibiotics.

### Can a child become allergic to any antibiotic?

Yes. The common problems, however, are not allergies but undesirable side effects such as nausea, diarrhea or itching near the anus (rectum).

### Which antibiotics can cause allergies?

Penicillin and sulfa drugs cause most allergic problems. Penicillin, for example, is broken down into different chemicals in the body and a child can become allergic to one or more of these altered penicillin forms. Some children are allergic to several antibiotics. This can create major difficulties whenever they develop a severe infection. Theoretically, anyone could become allergic to any antibiotic but fortunately most people do not.

### What do you do if your child is allergic to penicillin (or horse serum) and this is the *only* drug which can help the illness?

Your physician will probably want to contact an allergist who may attempt to treat your child with it very cautiously. There are usually other drugs which would be equally effective.

### What is the significance of diarrhea caused by an antibiotic?

This usually means that the medicine is irritating the bowel. It does not mean that the patient will not be helped by the medicine because its effectiveness is determined by how much is absorbed and whether the drug will combat the infecting germs. It also does not mean that the patient is allergic to it. Diarrhea is a very common, undesirable side effect caused by many drugs. If it is mild, no special treatment is needed; if it is severe, your physician must be contacted.

### Do allergies to antibiotics tend to be found in families?

Yes. Sometimes several members of the same family are allergic to penicillin, for example. If this is noted, penicillin should not be prescribed for other members unless this is the *only* drug which would help the infection being treated. Aspirin sensitivity, associated with asthma, may also be found in families of very allergic persons. If one family member is allergic, use an aspirin substitute for the entire family.

It is not unusual for patients to believe they are allergic to a drug when in fact they are not. Check with your physician if you are not sure. Sometimes drug allergies subside when a drug is avoided for a long period of time.

# PART SIX

# Circumstances creating potential problems for allergic persons

THIS section realistically discusses many common yet difficult problems facing some allergic persons.

Chapter 15 concerns the thorny problem of pets, including what should be done when an allergic person has, wants, or needs a pet.

Chapter 16 explains the relatively uncommon problem of an allergy to a stinging insect and why this type of allergy is so serious. It describes a normal and abnormal reaction to a sting, tells exactly how each should be treated, how to avoid stings and the dangers of not securing proper treatment.

Chapter 17 anticipates the possible causes of allergy in the grade school (or college) situation. Gym, sports, cafeteria foods, parties and misunderstandings by many make allergies a special problem at school.

Chapter 18 covers the common problems of the allergic child at camp. If your child is well prepared and problems are anticipated, there should be less difficulty.

Chapter 19 gives some common causes of allergies during certain holidays.

Chapter 20 explains the specific difficulties facing a person who is traveling and allergic to common items such as dust or certain foods. The difficulty related to receiving an allergy-extract injection while en route is also discussed.

# CHAPTER 15

# *Pets*

### Which pets cause allergies?

Any animal with feathers or fur can cause difficulty. This would include cats, dogs, horses, hamsters, mice, rabbits, parakeets, gerbils, cattle, hogs, goats or chickens. It is not only the hair but also the dander or saliva which starts allergic symptoms. Cats and horses seem to cause more extreme symptoms than other pets.

The pet does not have to be in a room to cause symptoms. The hair and dander in the air, on the walls, in the carpets and on furniture can cause symptoms even after the pet is gone. Thorough cleaning, of course, helps. It has been stated that chihuahuas and poodles do not cause allergies because they do not shed. It has even been said that chihuahuas might help allergic children. This is quite untrue, as these dogs do have dander and can cause allergic symptoms.

### Which pets do *not* cause allergies?

Pets which do not have fur or feathers, such as fish, turtles, snakes or alligators. On rare occasions, children who are very allergic to fish can have symptoms from contact with pet fish. Fish food or algae are rare problems.

### Which allergic symptoms do pets cause?

They can cause any type of allergic symptoms; however, chest (asthma or cough), eye, nose or skin reactions are the most common. The skin manifestations could be eczema, hives, or itching. Hyperactivity and behavior problems are possible but not common.

### How can children who are allergic to rabbits avoid them?

In addition to avoiding the animal, remember to have your child avoid rabbits' feet or rabbit-trimmed clothing. Do not allow your child to wear gloves lined with rabbit fur or fur-trimmed coats. It is possible but unlikely that a mother's fur-trimmed coat could cause symptoms. Felt can be made from rabbit fur, as can bedding, upholstery or drapery material.

### How can horse-sensitive children avoid these animals?

If your child is allergic to horses or ponies, he should avoid horsehair blankets or mattresses as well as stables and contact with another person's riding clothes. Avoid furniture filled with rubberized horsehair, found in some chairs or couches.

If your child has only a slight reaction to horsehair, and has no obvious symptoms of allergies when he's near a horse, he may occasionally ride one at a fair or when the family is on vacation. Be certain, however, at those times to carry the appropriate allergy medicines, so that they can be given if necessary.

### How can feathers be avoided by children allergic to them?

Avoid birds and feather or down pillows. Avoid feather-filled sleeping bags, comforters, quilts or any feather-filled furniture. Also avoid Indian headdresses and feather dusters.

### What is the significance of a positive or negative skin test for a pet?

A positive skin test usually indicates an allergy to the pet for which the child was tested and a negative test means there is no allergy. These tests are not, however, always accurate or completely reliable because the allergist uses a stock dog extract. It is possible that this was made, for example, from cocker spaniel hair and dander, while your child may be allergic to some other breed of dog.

It is possible to be allergic only to your own dog, without necessarily being allergic to other dogs of that breed or any other breed.

### Can your child be given allergy-extract treatments for pet allergies?

Yes, but these may not be helpful and may precipitate nasal and chest allergies because the animal extracts are highly potent. Most allergists recommend avoidance of the animal rather than allergy-extract injections. Allpyral and aqueous animal extracts have been helpful in treating some children. Treatment with the ''correct'' dosage after titration testing is also sometimes effective.

### When are patients treated with extracts of animals?

This is a necessity if the pet exposure is occupational, as with a veterinarian or a furrier, or if the patient is employed as a laboratory worker where animals cannot be avoided. Children do not usually have to receive treatments unless their family raises animals which the child could not possibly avoid. Sometimes a pet allergy decreases when the patient is successfully treated for allergies.

**Can someone be allergic to a pet even though no obvious symptoms are noted when playing with the animal?**

Yes. If the sensitivity is mild, symptoms might not be evidenced unless the child's allergy threshold has been exceeded. A combination of house dust plus cat hair may cause symptoms whereas either alone may not (see pp. 19-20). A cat which is shedding dander and hair may cause symptoms at that time, but not ordinarily. Touching the cat's fur may not cause symptoms, but if the cat were to lick the face of a child allergic to its saliva, a definite allergic reaction could occur. Symptoms can be caused by even the slightest contact with pets if the sensitivity is very great. Remember that a reaction may not occur immediately. A child could play with a cat in the afternoon and not wheeze till late at night or during the night. Every allergist has patients who were certain that the family pet was not related to their allergies. Their symptoms, however, subsided shortly after the death or removal of their pet.

**What will happen if a child knows that he is definitely allergic to his pet and yet refuses to part with it?**

Allergic symptoms will continue. They may also become more severe or more frequently noted the longer the pet is kept. Children need love and understanding which at times only a pet can furnish. It is indeed unfortunate that physicians have not been able as yet to devise extracts which are entirely safe and helpful in relieving pet sensitivities. If the pet's departure from the home will cause more emotional difficulty than the allergy symptoms, then the pet could stay for a trial period. The following may decrease the problem:

1. Keep the pet outside all the time if possible.

2. Or confine the pet to the basement or possibly the kitchen, but *never* allow it in the bedrooms or on the furniture. Never let a child lie on the carpet if the pet is allowed in that room.

3. Have the child wash his hands after contact with the pet. A mask might also help, for example, when cleaning a pet's cage. Whenever possible, grooming and care of a pet should be done by someone other than the allergic person. Discourage contact between the child and pet as much as possible.

4. Connect an electronic air-purifier to the furnace or at least use portable units in the rooms where the pet is allowed. This will decrease air contamination.

5. Spray your dog with Allergex.

6. Try therapy using the bioassay titration end-point method and see if it helps.

### What happens when an allergic child with a negative skin reaction to a pet keeps it confined to the outside or basement and avoids close contact?

On repeated skin-testing these children may remain skin-test negative to the pet. If, however, the pet is allowed in the bedroom "occasionally" or in the family room, the test frequently changes from negative to positive or becomes more positive within one or two years. Every allergist has seen patients do this. The previously well controlled child begins to have more and more symptoms because of the pet, and the entire situation becomes impossible. It is not fair to keep pets outside in many areas because of the bad weather or traffic.

### If your child is allergic and your present pet dies, should you acquire another?

No. Not if you truly want to do everything you can to keep your child well. Pets and allergies do not mix. If you are given a pet, return it while it is young enough to be wanted in another home.

### If your child is allergic, but not to pets, when can you acquire a pet?

A definite answer cannot be given. If your sole concern is for the health of your child, no pet should be acquired until allergists can more certainly and safely treat for pet allergies.

If a pet is acquired, sensitivity to it can occur at any time. It could happen in weeks or months, or might take years before problems were noted. It is also possible that no pet allergy would ever occur. Remember, if you get a pet and your child develops symptoms whenever the pet is touched, it is not easy to remove the pet. Pets are often loved like children and one cannot just give them away or destroy them. Other children in the family will resent the one child's allergy, as this has deprived them of the animal which was so loved and wanted. It is not pleasant to choose between the health of one child and the happiness of the family.

### If your child is allergic, how can you visit relatives who have pets?

There is no easy solution. Have the relatives visit you as much as possible. Urge them not to hold the pet on their laps and then come to your home and put your child there, as this could cause symptoms. If you want to visit relatives during holidays, then the pet should, if possible, be confined to an area of the home which the allergic child could avoid. The rest of the home should be thoroughly cleaned to eliminate the animal's dander and hair. Prior to the visit, the child should be given the appropriate medicines to prevent allergic symptoms and these medicines should be continued prophylactically during the entire visit.

If the stay is to be prolonged, carry your child's own pillows, blankets, a barrier-cloth mattress cover, and possibly a portable de-pollution unit. If the symptoms become severe, you may have to stay in a motel.

It is certainly a great inconvenience to any relative to ask that all this be done before bringing your child to visit. It might be wiser and easier to ask relatives to your allergy-free home. Also give asthmatics Intal before and during the visit.

### Can visiting the zoo cause symptoms of allergies?

Yes. Again, this is related to how similar the pets are to the ones which cause the children's sensitivity. The lion house could cause difficulty for a patient allergic to cats.

Walking outside the zoo house would cause difficulty in some sensitive children. Inside the animal house, the hair and dander could easily exceed the tolerated amount and would cause potential difficulty in more children. To solve this problem, if you are uncertain, visit the animals kept outside and carry the proper medicine with you. If you notice any symptoms, give the appropriate medicine. If there is no difficulty outside the animal houses, then you could try going inside. If any problems are noted, immediately leave and use the appropriate medicines, if they have not already been given.

If your child's class is planning a visit to the zoo, you should accompany them or make a preliminary visit with your child to see if it causes any difficulty. Be certain the teacher in charge has the appropriate medicines to use if your youngster develops symptoms.

### What other contacts with animals can cause symptoms?

Children allergic to animals or birds should avoid enclosed bird sanctuaries, circuses, bullfights, dog, cat, and horse shows, racetracks, farms, or county fairs. Fish-sensitive patients may have difficulty at "marine" shows.

# CHAPTER 16

# *Insect problems*

**Which insects cause allergies?**

Bees, wasps, hornets, yellow jackets, scorpions and caterpillars are the major causes of stings. In the southern United States, biting ants are a problem. Other biting insects include deer, horse and black flies, midges, bedbugs, kissing bugs, fleas, lice and spiders.

**Do mosquito bites cause allergy?**

Mosquito bites often cause extreme swelling in young children but this becomes less of a problem as the child ages. Such reactions usually do not require allergy-injection therapy, although this is possible. Vitamin $B_1$, or thiamine hydrochloride, in daily doses of 75 to 150 mg. is said to repel mosquitoes in some patients. A paste of meat tenderizer and water often relieves the itching.

We do not understand why mosquitoes or other stinging insects seem to be attracted to some people.

Treatment for mosquito sensitivity using the bioassay titration endpoint method is claimed by some physicians to be effective.

**What is an "abnormal" or severe reaction to a sting which could indicate an allergic reaction?**

The local reaction does not remain in the area of the sting. Thus, if the sting was on the arm, the swelling may involve more than the arm. Often, there is swelling of several parts of the body, or hives and itching all over the body. Sometimes children develop asthma, hay fever, a tight throat, an intestinal upset, have to move their bowels or urinate, or feel dizzy and become unconscious. This type of reaction means your child should be seen by a physician immediately. It is a "severe" reaction. Your child must also wear a name tag stating that he has this type of allergy.

Some elderly patients die of apparent heart failure when they are stung. Many people have extremely severe local reactions to a sting and some of these patients do have an allergy which can be detected by the RAST test.

## How can you identify stinging insects?

It is not easy. Wasps have no hair and have a tiny "wasp" waist. They nest in open paper or mud combs under eaves, on porches, in sheds, etc. Hornets and yellow jackets are both hairy and can be black and yellow. They are easily confused with wasps. Hornets have football-shaped, papier-mâché-like nests hanging in trees, from bushes or on houses, usually under the eaves. Honeybees are small and are very common in garden areas, hollows in trees, in cracks or under boards in houses. Yellow jackets nest in the ground, under stones or between walls. Bumblebees also nest underground. Barefoot children are very frequently stung by these ground-nesting insects. In case of a sting which causes trouble, save the insect and show it to your allergist, if possible. Only honeybees leave their stingers in their victims.

## Are children who have allergies more apt to have reactions to stinging insects?

These reactions occur in persons who have no allergies in the family, as well as those who do. Serious reactions, however, do appear to be somewhat more common in patients who have strong allergies.

## What is a "normal" reaction to an insect sting?

All stings cause swelling, pain and itching in the stung area. If the sting is on the face, normally the eyes or lips will swell greatly. The reaction should remain localized to the area of the sting and not affect the rest of the body.

## What is a toxic reaction to a stinging insect?

This could be manifested by swelling without hives, by headache, fever, drowsiness, weakness, muscle spasm or even convulsions. At times it may be difficult to tell the difference between a toxic and an allergic reaction. Toxic reactions usually occur when a child is stung by many bees at once because each bee injects a little toxin. This toxin is an insect poison harmful to the human body.

## What is a delayed reaction to an insect sting?

These reactions occur in about 24 hours or up to one week or ten days after a sting. This is in sharp contrast to the almost immediate reaction which is noted after most allergic stings. The delayed reactions can include fever, swelling, joint problems, hives or bleeding, or neurological problems such as headache or dizziness. Only about two per cent of all stinging insect reactions are of the delayed type. Some patients have both an immediate and a delayed reaction.

## What immediate treatment should you give for an insect sting?

Any child will be better if:

1. The stinger is removed very gently. It is dark and looks like a tiny matchhead. Only honeybees leave their stinger imbedded in a victim's skin. The stinger is often attached to a sac of venom and, when the stinger is removed, you must be careful not to squeeze the sac or you could force more venom into the child's skin. Flick it out using a fingernail.

2. Apply ice to the area of the sting.

3. Apply Calamine lotion with phenol (no prescription needed) if the area of the sting is itchy, or apply a paste of meat tenderizer and water.

4. Aspirin (or an aspirin substitute such as Tylenol) helps to reduce pain. Don't use aspirin if there is an allergy to it.

If your child has previously had or seems to be having an allergic reaction to the sting, also do the following:

5. Apply a tourniquet, using a shoestring or any other means, if an extremity is involved. This should be released for a few seconds every ten to 15 minutes.

6. Give your child an antihistamine, such as Triaminic, and an anti-asthmatic medicine if these are available. An epinephrine-like inhaler could immediately help to prevent breathing problems and should be used if asthma or difficulty in speaking occurs, *unless* epinephrine by injection can immediately be given.

7. If there is a severe reaction (see above), an injection of Adrenalin is indicated. This can be obtained from your physician, or at the nearest hospital if you are not carrying a kit which contains epinephrine (Adrenalin).

8. Cortisone or steroids are not very helpful immediately since they may require hours before they have a noticeable benefit. They are sometimes prescribed to relieve or diminish persistent itching or swelling.

9. Keep the insect sting area clean. Secondary infection resulting from scratching with dirty fingernails can sometimes require a physician's advice.

## If your child has been well treated for stinging-insect allergies, what should you do when he is stung?

You should carefully remove the stinger and apply ice, Calamine, or a paste of meat tenderizer to the area. An antihistamine and an asthma medicine should probably also be given unless your child was previously stung after treatments were started and had no reaction other than local swelling and slight pain. If for some reason you are concerned, have a physician examine your child or take him to the nearest hospital. About 90 per cent of well treated patients usually have no problems with insect stings while they are being given extract injections.

### Can insect stings be fatal?

Yes. For this reason, treatment by an allergist after an abnormal or severe allergic reaction to stinging insects is vitally important. The patient may have only 10 to 15 minutes. If the sting causes no adverse effects within 30 minutes, chances are excellent that no problems will arise. Stings in the area of the neck are especially dangerous.

### Does skin testing help to diagnose insect allergy?

Yes. The allergist will try to identify which insect is causing a reaction. Often stinging insects are so similar that the child may be sensitive to more than one, although only one type has stung the child. Skin testing for stinging insects is most accurate if it is done two weeks or longer after the sting, because there may be a refractory period when tests would not be reliable. Tests with pure venom are more reliable than those done with whole insect-body extract. Newer blood tests (RAST) are easy and accurate in the detection of this kind of allergy.

### Does allergy-injection treatment help stinging-insect allergy?

Yes. Once a patient is adequately treated, much less difficulty is noted with subsequent stings, or perhaps none at all. Injection treatments are about 95 per cent effective. Because there is a similarity among stinging insects, a combination of bee, wasp, yellow jacket and hornet extract is customarily used for treatment. Therapy for a single insect sting is used if the patient is allergic to the particular type of insect.

### Can you predict if a child might have a bad reaction to an insect sting?

Not always. Only about 50 per cent of children who are going to have a severe allergic reaction to a sting will have had a previous reaction which was extreme or unusual. Such warnings should not be neglected because the next sting could be fatal. One such warning would be hives on an area of the body other than in the region of the actual sting.

Many parents worry that their child might have an allergic reaction to a stinging insect at some future time. Be assured, most children do not have unusual reactions to insect stings, but if one does unexpectedly happen to your child, give him an antihistamine and asthma medicine, if these are available, and follow the recommendations on page 237. If you are concerned for some specific reason, a RAST test can be performed.

### For how many years should a child receive stinging-insect allergy treatments?

In the past it was recommended that treatments be continued indefinitely. It is now possible to study the patient's blood serum by doing a RAST test and from this one can tell if the patient continues to be allergic and also if adequate protection against stinging insects is present in the blood. At present, this test is readily available for only certain types of stinging insects.

### If a child has stinging-insect allergy, and is untreated, how much time may elapse between the sting and a possible severe fatal reaction?

Usually only a few minutes, 10 or 15, or less than an hour. This is why parents and patients *must be* prepared. You may not have time to secure medical help. On rare occasions persons have died several days after an insect sting.[1]

### How can you protect your child from insect stings?

1. Don't allow your child to wear flowers, use scented hair or skin preparations, or wear any gaily colored or flowered clothing or bright metal jewelry. Insects can become confused. Tan, white or green smooth-surfaced clothing should be worn rather than dark-colored or flower-patterned, rough fabrics. Discourage your child from walking barefoot or wearing sandals outdoors because insects can nest in the ground or be near clover in lawns.

2. Have your child use an insect repellent such as OFF liquid on his hair and clothing. Thiamine hydrochloride (vitamin $B_1$), given in a 75- to 150-mg daily dose, is said to repel insects. Keep an insect spray repellent in your car and near the child's bed. Do not use these if chemical odors cause symptoms.

3. Have your child carry a chewable anthihistamine (Tacaryl) and asthma medicine *at all times* if he had an abnormal reaction to an insect

---

[1] Due to the urgency for immediate therapy, many state laws exempt teachers and school personnel from liability when they administer emergency treatment to allergic persons. If your child has a stinging-insect problem, ask if the teacher will learn to give an injection of epinephrine and supply her with an emergency kit.

but is not as yet adequately treated for stinging insects. Also have the stinging-insect kit (prepared by Hollister-Stier and available on prescription from your druggist) in your car and at home for emergency use (and recommend it for school use). This kit contains a syringe filled with epinephrine, a tourniquet, an asthma medicine, and an antihistamine. Children under 40 pounds should receive no more than 0.1 or 0.15 cc of 1-1000 Adrenalin in the prefilled syringe. Check with your physician about the dose your child should receive. It should be colorless. Replace the Adrenalin if it turns brown. Check the kit on occasion to be certain the medicine has not leaked from the syringe. Keep this handy in your car.

4. Have your child avoid bushes, gardens, lawns covered with clover, old trees, eaves of houses and attics. Beware in particular of any struggling stinging insect on the surface of a swimming pool. Such insects often sting. Don't permit your child to tamper with insect nests.

5. Your child should wear a name tag stating that he has a stinging-insect allergy.

6. Exterminate stinging insect nests near your home. Local beekeepers often will help remove honeybees. The odor of gasoline, kerosene or ammonia poured down the holes of yellow jackets at night will kill them. Fill the hole with dirt after you do this.

### What is the current status of stinging-insect treatment?

Currently it is believed that treatment with whole-body stinging extract vaccine is not as effective as treatment with pure venom. The major problem at present is that pure venom for each type of stinging insect is in short supply and the cost is exorbitant. Perhaps bioassay titration stinging-insect therapy will be seriously considered to help resolve this problem. It might afford an effective but inexpensive method to treat susceptible patients, but it will be years before studies to investigate these methods can be conducted.

Newer testing methods can tell which patients are in potential danger because of their stinging-insect allergy and also if they have had sufficient treatment to protect them from a sting. Ask your physician about RAST tests for stinging insects.

### Can a stinging-insect allergy make a young man ineligible for the armed service?

A severe or moderate, generalized reaction to a stinging insect can medically disqualify a young man for service in the armed forces. A physician's statement concerning the details of the reaction would be required.

# CHAPTER 17

# *Allergies related to school*

**Do children have more allergies at home or at school?**

Most children have fewer allergy problems at school than they do at home because homes contain many more substances capable of causing allergies. However, modern, carpeted schools filled with synthetic, odorous items may alter this situation.

**Which classes in school cause difficulty for allergic children?**

Special classes often require the use of special substances for certain projects and many of these could cause symptoms of allergy.

The following situations could be troublesome:

ART CLASS—dried flowers, leaves or plant life, use of clay, kilns and glaze paints, wallpaper paste, glue, rubber cement, tempera or water-color paint, crayons, cellophane, construction paper, india and linoleum inks or marking pencils and pens. Aerosol sprays can be especially bad.

COOKING CLASS—smells of such foods as nuts, eggs, potatoes, fish or flour. Colored sweet beverages can be a problem.

CLASSROOMS—any animals with fur or feathers, chalk, teachers' or children's cosmetics, perfumes, hair sprays or after-shaving lotions; any printed or mimeograph paper, stencils or chemically impregnated copy paper causing an odor, flowers (artificial or real), molds, carpets or carpet pads.

CHEMISTRY CLASS—the chemicals used in odors or fumes from experiments.

GYM CLASS—locker rooms and gym floors or mats can be dusty, musty or moldy. New rubber composition floors may cause offensive odors. Outdoor gym classes expose children to various pollens and mold spores during the warm months and when it is colder the cool air can precipitate asthmatic attacks. Leaves in the fall are moldy, as is most outside vegetation.

PRINTING CLASS—the smell of the ink or contact with it could cause symptoms in children allergic to flaxseed.

WOODWORKING OR METAL SHOP—the smells of paint-thinners, rubber cement, sawdust, lacquers, shellacs, paints, plastics, smoke or air pollutants.

### How does one handle the gym problem for the asthmatic child?

The answer is to use common sense.

If gym causes no conspicuous difficulty, the child should participate in the customary manner. If gym causes symptoms, the child should try to take medicine such as Intal for asthma about ten minutes before his gym class. A note from your physician will be required for this. If medicines for asthma are taken before gym and your child wheezes in spite of this medication, this activity must be discontinued. If your child starts to take gym and suddenly feels short of breath or begins to have trouble breathing, he should be allowed to stop immediately and take the proper medication. Some children are shy about complaining or are ashamed of taking medicines. The gym teacher should be informed so that this child can be watched more closely and advised to stop if any symptoms of allergy are noted. Other children tend to use their allergies as a cover for their dislike of gym, showers or swimming. For example, pubescent girls often resent communal showers and early- or late-maturing boys may avoid nude swimming. Your physician may have to help solve these problems.

### May allergic children enter competitive sports?

Surely; but if they wheeze, their performance will probably be better if they use asthma medication prior to actual participation to help their lung capacity to be more normal. Antihistamines should be avoided before participation in competitive sports because they often cause poor coordination and sleepiness.

### Does swimming cause special problems?

It can. Children are rarely allergic to chlorine, although if the pool is heavily chlorinated, this can be an irritant and aggravate allergies, especially in the nose or eyes. Some pools smell musty and this could precipitate symptoms in mold-sensitive patients. Algae in some pools could also be the cause of asthma or skin rashes.

If a child is required to leave school, for some reason, immediately after gym, this could enhance the chances of his developing a cold. Hair is frequently wet after swimming and, if the child is not properly attired, exposure to bad weather could trigger allergic symptoms or infection. Children with eczema are not adversely affected although they may often swim for prolonged periods of time in chlorinated pools.

Strong soaps used when showering after swimming, however, could further dry the child's skin. Scented items in the shower room might cause symptoms. Asthmatics tolerate swimming better than other sports.

### Do school parties cause problems in allergic children?

Yes. Often a birthday-child brings cakes or cookies for the entire class and, unless the mother of the food-allergic child provides a suitable substitute, eggs, milk, chocolate, nuts or nut-flavoring could cause trouble. Try potato chips without additives and a colorless diet beverage. Easter, Halloween and Christmas parties can be a challenge for food-allergic children.

### Will your child feel "left out" if gym cannot be taken or if special consideration must be given at party time or during eating periods?

Yes, unfortunately this can be the case unless the gym instructor, teacher, principal and school nurse are all sympathetic and aware of the situation. Many times, children are made the butt of ridicule by unknowing persons who feel the allergic child's problems are "all emotional." It is hoped that parents and physicians will be able to inform school authorities to the point where they will understand and help, as only they can, in such a situation.

Particularly upsetting is the practice in some schools which forces children who have allergies to sit on the sidelines and watch the other children having fun in gym. This is akin to asking these children to watch while you give ice cream to everyone except them. Special provisions should be made so that these children are allowed to go to a study room or library during this period of time.

### Can school cafeteria food cause allergic symptoms?

Children who have severe food allergies should carry their lunches, because lunchtime can prove a major challenge and a constant threat. Eating dyed sweet foods or beverages, eggs, milk, potatoes, wheat, pork, certain spices, tomatoes, fish and chocolate can readily cause difficulty. Odors of nuts or fish also can precipitate symptoms. Meals that contain a speck of the food to which a child is sensitive can, if eaten, cause immediate and at times alarming symptoms of a wide variety. These include itching or swelling of the mouth, lips or throat, or asthma, hay fever or a digestive problem. A child innocently sharing an almond-flavored cookie or offering a bite of a peanut butter sandwich can cause grave problems for the youngster allergic to nuts. Lunch swapping is common and must be discouraged. (Refer to page 271 for lists of foods often unexpectedly containing milk, or wheat, and eggs.)

## What particular problems do allergic children have in nursery school or kindergarten?

1. Children frequently sleep on the floor during nap time. Children allergic to dust should not do this; if it is necessary, be sure that the sleeping mat or towel is laundered between uses.

2. Little children frequently are sent to school when they have slight infections, and they tend to cough or sneeze without covering their faces. Because of this increased exposure many children have frequent colds during the first year of school. In asthmatic children, infections usually trigger asthma attacks. This can frequently be aborted or prevented by vigorous treatment of the asthma and the infection at its earliest sign.

3. Nursery schools often have party foods which cause difficulty for children allergic to eggs, milk or nuts. The younger the child, the more likely foods are liable to be a factor related to allergic symptoms. Dyed or sweet foods or beverages can cause hyperactivity in some children.

4. Nursery schools often have pets in the classroom which can cause trouble for allergic children.

5. Handling clay, fingerpaints or putty-like substances causes problems for some children.

## Why are responsible, educated, intelligent adults (often medically trained) not allowed to give medicine in schools to children in emergencies?

Most states have laws which permit a child to receive medicine only *at specific times,* when the medicines are labeled and exact instructions have been supplied by a physician. No provision, however, is made for giving allergy medicines on a discretionary or emergency basis. The interpretation of the law by some school officials is such that teachers or nurses are forbidden to make a value judgment or use discretion about giving medications in medical emergencies. Teachers are certainly not trained to do this but should have enough judgment to call the nurse, if the school has one. The nurse must, in turn, decide whether the parents or a physician should be called. Some discretion is therefore required and used. Some schools do not have full-time principals to make final decisons when these are necessary.

From the teacher's viewpoint, it certainly is not fair to ask her to give medicine to a wheezing child while a whole class of anxious students is "trying to help." If she gives the medicine to one child, will she eventually be asked to control a medicine cabinet full of drugs for a number of children?

From the allergic child's viewpoint, emergencies are simply going to arise, try as one may to avoid them. Let us suppose that a child is very allergic to nuts. If someone puts almond extract in a cake frosting and the child eats it in the cafeteria, his lips swell immediately, he is covered with hives, his eyes water and swell, his nose runs and he is having severe difficulty breathing because of swelling of his upper air tubes (larynx). There may be little time to call the physician or family, or they may not be available. The school has an allergy medicine that is not dangerous to give in a single dose in such a situation, and the dose is clearly labeled. Why can't the medicine be given? In some schools no one wants to take the responsibility and legally no one has to. If such a situation should happen to your child, you should check the laws in your state to see if he could be treated immediately and on an emergency basis.

The solution to such a problem is not an easy one but there are times for exceptions and times when each of us has to answer only to himself. We may hope that legislators eventually will allow registered school nurses to be in fact nurses. We may hope that schools for training teachers will prepare them to handle temporary medical emergencies and that states which have laws to protect schools eventually will appreciate the plight of the allergic child.

### Should your child ride a school bus?

Yes, if walking the distance between home and school causes symptoms of allergies. Your physician can provide the necessary permit requesting this. Medicine given just before leaving home and again just before school closes may help.

Some school buses have noxious fumes or permit smoking, which could possibly precipitate chest or nasal allergic symptoms.

In winter, cold air frequently triggers symptoms. Breathing with the lips closed or covering the mouth with a scarf may cause air to reach the lungs more slowly. This gives the respiratory system a chance to warm the air before it arrives in the lungs, thereby lessening the chance of lung spasm from the cold air.

### Can fire drills aggravate allergies in some children?

They can certainly precipitate symptoms because children often do not wear their coats, and slight chilling, at times, can start wheezing or infection in asthmatic children. Anticipate this problem and obtain a note from your physician.

### Should a wheezing child be sent to school?

The answer depends upon whether this is "normal" for your child. If your youngster always wheezes a little and is controlled by daily medicine, by all means allow school attendance. If, however, your child could not sleep all night because of wheezing or coughing, or suddenly seems to have repeated episodes of asthma, something is wrong and your child should be examined thoroughly by your physician in an effort to determine the cause of the problem.

Under no circumstances should you allow your wheezing child to go to school merely because *he wants to go.* It is unfortunate that a youngster may have to miss a Halloween, Christmas, Valentine or birthday party, but your child's health is more important. If your child is most anxious to go to school but you feel it is unwise, do *not* allow him to go. If you are unsure, call your physician and he will help you make the right decision. Some asthmatics try to use their asthma as an excuse for not going to school.

### Do school heating systems cause allergies?

These can cause the same problems as in any home. Dust in forced hot-air systems and oil or gas odors can cause allergic symptoms.

### Can custodial care at school cause allergic symptoms?

Yes. Sweeping compounds and treated dust cloths could cause difficulty, as can cleaning supplies, aerosols,. waxes or polishes. Any chemical odor—insecticides, pesticides, fungicides—can cause symptoms in some children.

### What should you tell the school nurse and teacher about your child's allergies?

You can't ever give them too much information. It is important that both understand the child's problems as fully as possible because school nurses often work in more than one school, or a teacher may be absent. Both should know exactly which medicines must be given for certain symptoms. The school should have medicines clearly labeled with the name of the child, the dosage, and why and when it should be given. The child's physician can furnish this information. Be very careful that the school has the telephone number of your home, of the father's and mother's places of employment and of the child's physician, so that someone responsible can be contacted if a major problem arises. By law in some states, children are not allowed to carry their own medicines in school.

CHAPTER 18

# *Summer camp and the allergic child*

**Should children with allergies go to camp?**

It depends upon the child's allergy. If the patient has eczema, eye, ear or nasal allergies, camp should not be a significant problem provided that a nurse is there and the proper medicines are taken along. Unless some special problem exists, the camp does not need to be one specially selected for allergic children.

If the child has asthma which is not usually a severe or major problem, a camp with full-time medical personnel should be selected. A physician must be available for emergencies, and a nurse present at all times.

If a child has severe asthma, camp is not a safe place unless it is a camp specially adapted for allergic children. A camp of this type for both boys and girls, age six to 15, is Bronco Junction.

It is surprising how often pollen-allergic children do very well at camp after they have been treated with extract injections. If your child has special allergic problems, contact your allergist and obtain his advice regarding camp. Every effort should be made to allow children to camp whenever sensibly possible.

**What are the major potential sources of difficulty related to allergies at camps?**

ENVIRONMENT

Cabins are often dusty and old. Cleaning or sweeping the cabins is certain to precipitate symptoms in some allergic patients. Tents are often folded and packed away while damp, a condition which causes them to become moldy and aggravates allergies. Camp fires are a part of camp life and the irritating smoke can trigger both nasal and chest allergies. Urge your child to sit so that the smoke from the fire does not blow toward his face. Hiking and nature study are frequent activities and these would possibly expose children to pollens or other substances which cause allergies. Animals on campsites often cause symptoms in those children allergic to them. Children who have a slight sensitivity to horse dander or hair might be able to ride outdoors, but attempts to enter or work in the stables could trigger attacks. Other children are so allergic to horses that contact with someone else's riding clothing can cause symptoms. Allergic children should take their own bedding to camp. Their sleeping bags should be synthetic, never stuffed with down or kapok. They should never sleep on straw mattresses.

FOODS

If someone is allergic to a certain food, this again could create many problems in camp unless special consideration was given to the allergic child. The cook, for example, would have to know that many hot dogs or wieners contain milk or wheat products and these should not be given to children with these food sensitivities. This would be an unreasonable request to make at most camps. Persons unacquainted with allergies find it difficult to accept that the smell of a food, or even a speck of a certain food in something, can cause immediate reactions in persons allergic to the offending substances. So if a child has a significant food allergy, only a camp for allergic children should be considered.

MEDICINES

There should be personnel at the camp who can care for medical emergencies and give required medicines. If a camp accepts moderately or severely asthmatic children, it should have a full-time physician. A parent must be certain that his child takes an adequate supply of well labeled medicines to camp. Each medicine must bear the name of the patient, the identity and dosage of the medicine and its purpose. Your child's physician will provide this information. If a child has a stinging-insect problem, he must carry emergency asthma and hay fever medicine at all times and someone at camp must have epinephrine and a stinging-insect kit (see p. 287) so that this can be given. If your child is allergic to horse serum, be certain that his tetanus immunization is up-to-date prior to going to camp. Check to see that he wears his tag to warn against the use of horse serum.

ACTIVITIES

Any activity, in excess, can precipitate asthmatic symptoms. Children who wheeze with activity should be given medicine *before* they engage in vigorous play. They should be urged to stop playing if they notice breathing problems and to rest until they are better. If a certain activity repeatedly causes asthma, they should avoid that endeavor and engage in other forms of entertainment which cause fewer symptoms.

Swimming can cause difficulty in some children. Cold air or water can cause itching and hives, and can precipitate wheezing in some children. Some youngsters are so sensitive to cold water that they could become seriously ill if they jumped into a cold pool or stream because they could develop hives all over their body. This type of physical allergy is, fortunately, uncommon.

Children who have nasal and ear allergies should wear a nose mask or a nose clip when they are swimming. Diving and underwater swimming should be strongly discouraged. Children who have recurrent ear problems should wear greased woolen ear plugs or molds and bathing caps when they swim unless their ear specialist has specified no swimming.

Chlorine in water can irritate the eyes and noses of some children, especially if hay fever is a problem. (It is also possible to be allergic to the odor of chlorine in water but this would be a rare sensitivity and would be apparent mainly from drinking chlorinated water.) Algae in water have been reported to cause asthma and skin rashes in some children.

INFECTIONS

Many asthmatic children will wheeze with every infection. This can best be handled by immediately treating the infection and starting asthma medicine at the first sign of a cold or sore throat. Your child should be urged to notify a responsible adult as soon as a problem of this type arises.

## What can be done about the allergy-extract treatment that is due while a child is at camp?

Try to avoid the problem by obtaining the allergy-injection treatment the day before the child leaves for camp even if it is not due for two or three weeks (see p. 189). Most children are on a monthly schedule and may not be at camp this long. If the extract is due so often that it must be given at camp, the staff physician must have all details regarding the extract. These must include well labeled bottles with the child's name, extract name and strength and a slip telling the date by which the child must receive the injection. The exact amount and strength to be given must be specified (see p. 260). Be certain that the camp director realizes that your physician should be contacted (supply his name and phone number) if the camp doctor has any questions related to your child's extract or treatment. Try to prevent asthma at camp by using Intal prophylactically.

(continued on page 252)

SUMMER CAMPS FOR ASTHMATIC CHILDREN

| Location | Name | Director |
|---|---|---|
| *California* | | |
| Stanford | Camp Wheez | Joann Blessing, M.D.<br>Childrens Hospital<br>Stanford, Palo Alto, CA 94305 |
| Running Springs | Camp SCAMP[1,2] | Peter Kozak, M.D.<br>Lung Association of Orange County<br>1717 North Broadway<br>Santa Ana, CA 92706 |
| Running Springs | Asthma and Allergy Foundation<br>of America | Roger M. Katz, M.D.<br>Boys' Club #365 Campsite<br>Running Springs, CA 92382 |
| | The Los Angeles Lung<br>Association Asthma Camp[1] | Larry Robinson, M.D. |
| | The San Diego County Lung<br>Association | William Wallace, M.D. |
| *Florida* | | |
| Melrose | Camp Sunshine Station<br>(Lake Swan Camp)[2] | Dennis Spangler, M.D.<br>Florida Lung Association<br>P.O. Box 8127<br>Jacksonville, FL 32211 |
| *Minnesota* | | |
| 1820 Portland Avenue | Camp Superkids[1,2] | Richard T. Cushing, M.D. |

| Location | Camp | Contact |
|---|---|---|
| Chappaqua | (Day Camp)[2] | American Lung Association of Mid-New York, Inc. <br> 23 South Street <br> Utica, NY 13501 |
| | Wagon Road Camp[2] | 200 S. Broadway <br> Tarrytown, NY 10591 |
| *Oregon* <br> Colton | Camp Christmas Seal (Camp Colton) | John D. Minor, M.D. <br> Oregon Lung Association <br> 1020 S. W. Taylor <br> Suite 830 <br> Portland, OR 97205 |
| *Virginia* <br> Charlottesville | Holiday Trails[2] | Elsa Paulson, M.D. <br> Department of Pediatrics <br> University of Virginia <br> Charlottesville, VA 22904 |
| *Washington* <br> Seattle | Children's Orthopedic Hospital and Medical Center Camp[2] | S. J. Stamm, M.D. <br> 4800 Sandpoint Way, N.E. <br> Seattle, WA 98105 |
| *West Virginia* <br> R.D. #1 <br> Red House, WV 25168 | Bronco Junction[1,2] | Chandra M. Kumar, M.D. <br> Merie S. Scherr, M.D. <br> Allergy Rehabilitation Foundation, Inc. <br> 810 Atlas Building <br> Charleston, WV 25301 |

[1] Some scholarships available.
[2] Takes only state residents.

**Are special summer camps available for asthmatic children?**

Yes. The preceding is a list of camps (although it does not constitute an endorsement). Additional information about these or other camps can be obtained from the Asthma and Allergy Foundation of America. The age of children accepted ranges from six to 16 and camp lasts from five days to eight weeks, depending upon the one selected.

**How do you select the "best" time to send your allergic child to camp?**

Try to pick a time of the year when your child has the fewest allergic symptoms or send him to a camp where the pollens to which he is sensitive are not prevalent. In the northeastern United States, if molds are not a problem (while grasses and weeds are), send your child to camp from mid-July through early August. (See pages 278–281 for the pollination times in various parts of the United States.)

**How can you determine where pollen-free vacation areas are located?**

Write for the booklet *Hay Fever Holiday* from the Asthma and Allergy Foundation of America, 19 West 44th St., New York, N.Y. 10036.

**Can any child become allergic to poison ivy?**

Yes, anyone can. Often children are not allergic to it until after the age of six. Poison ivy is one of the most allergenic substances to which one can be exposed. It has been speculated that about 50 per cent of all people are allergic to it. Direct contact with any part of the plant, including the roots, can cause exposure to the allergy-producing sap. Indirect contact from burning the plant or petting a dog who had contact with it can also produce symptoms. Persons sensitive to poison ivy can develop a rash from cashew nut oil.

**What is characteristic about a poison-ivy rash?**

The rash is red, and water blisters, ranging in size from very tiny to extremely large, are usually noted. These are very itchy and, because of the patient's tendency to scratch, will often appear in rows or streaks. The fluid in the blister is not contagious. Scratching spreads the sap which causes the rash. Swelling, or edema, of the affected skin areas is not unusual. Exposed body areas, or those contaminated by sap on the child's hands, are mainly affected. The rash appears six to 24 hours after contact and, regardless of what is done, tends to last about two weeks. Treatment can help to keep the rash under control. Many patients also have a slight fever and feel tired.

### Should the skin be washed?

If your child is known to have had contact with poison ivy, it is helpful at times to thoroughly scrub the skin, clean the hair and shoes and change all clothing within two hours. An alcohol rinse is also helpful but this should not be used on the genitals. If the rash is already evident, the other skin areas should be thoroughly cleaned.

Under ordinary conditions swimming would not be prohibited unless the blisters were very large or the child was very uncomfortable. Try *not* to break the blisters. They will disappear if left alone.

### How should poison ivy be treated?

If it is mild you can apply Calamine lotion with phenol and have your child use an antihistamine until he can be seen by a dermatologist or allergist. Cortisone skin medicines, tablets and/or injections might be indicated depending upon the extent and severity of the skin rash. The rash can be slight one day and severe the next, so a physician should be consulted. If the skin area is swollen and oozing, it helps if wet packs are placed on the affected areas for half an hour at least four times a day. Domeboro™ packets or tablets (one dissolved in a pint of water) is an effective preparation that requires no prescription.

### How should it *not* be treated?

No person who has a poison-ivy rash should receive poison-ivy allergy-injection treatments until the rash is gone. Some physicians using titration testing might relieve symptoms by using the "correct" dose while the rash is present.

### What is the best possible treatment for poison ivy?

Prevention by knowing exactly what the plant looks like and instructing your child to avoid it.

### Who should receive allergy-protection treatments for poison ivy?

Only those children who cannot possibly avoid it and find that it is a serious, recurrent problem. There are two forms of treatment. One is by repeated injections and the other by taking a relatively inexpensive poison-ivy solution by mouth (obtainable through your physician from Hollister-Stier Laboratories). Gradually stronger and larger amounts of poison ivy are given to the patient by either method. The treatments are often inadvisable because sometimes they are not helpful and frequently cause a poison-ivy rash when attempts are made to increase the dose or strength of the poison-ivy medicine. The treatments must be given yearly and started at least two months before the time of possible exposure. Titration end-point therapy is not documented as effective but may enable a patient to have inexpensive, rapid relief of symptoms.

## How can you identify poison ivy?

Look for three leaflets in a compound leaf. The plant usually grows along the ground but can also grow like a vine or shrub. At times, it climbs the sides of trees or walls. The leaves are often shiny and, when very young, they may be reddish in color. In late summer the plant bears round, white berries. Characteristically, on one or both sides of the leaf there is often, but not always, a right-angle cut.

## How can you eliminate poison ivy on your property?

Contact a nursery and use broad-leaf herbicide preparations, such as Kill Brush (2,4,5 D), Amitrole or Ammate, as directed. All parts of the plant can cause a rash, including the roots. Be very careful when handling and disposing of the plants.

# CHAPTER 19

# Holiday allergies

**What are special problems related to Easter?**

Mainly these are centered on difficulties in eating chocolate, nuts in chocolate or eggs. Colored chocolate can cause the same symptoms as ordinary chocolate. Some mothers have noted that certain brands of chocolate cause allergic symptoms while others do not. Some chocolate has almond flavoring and this can cause symptoms in children allergic to nuts. Some children can tolerate hard-boiled eggs but not partially or less well cooked eggs. The dyes, spices or flavoring in certain jelly beans or candy coatings can cause trouble. Licorice is in the legume family, which contains peanuts, and some children allergic to peanuts would have difficulty with this flavor. Sugar and food coloring, in particular, cause hyperactivity in some children.

**What are special Halloween problems?**

The types of candy mentioned above can cause difficulty. Unless candy is well labeled it must not be eaten by children allergic to nuts. Sprayed apples that are not adequately washed or candied applies (with cinnamon) can create problems.

Some children have symptoms when they wear plastic masks with a chemical smell. The biggest problem related to Halloween is the fact that it is often damp and wet outdoors and children tend to become chilled and develop infections shortly after their night out for "tricks or treats."

**What special problems are related to Christmas?**

Evergreen trees can cause symptoms, although the reason for this is not clear. Some children have difficulty that starts the day the tree is put up and continues until it is removed. This can occur without touching the tree and is unrelated to the common, contact-type rash which these trees can cause. If this is noted, try an artificial tree. Some children seem to be able to tolerate some types of evergreens but not others, e.g., firs but not spruces, or vice versa. Some develop symptoms as soon as they enter a forest area where the family intends to cut down a tree. This could possibly be caused by the pine odor or molds on the evergreens. Terpine therapy might help.

Since some trees are color-sprayed, the odor of the dye could cause certain children to have symptoms.

Some parents forget that their child is allergic to trees and decorate with Christmas tree branches, or spray with an evergreen or pine scent. Incense or perfumed candles may also cause symptoms.

The worst problem remains the unavoidable exposure to evergreens. Though you may have banned them from your own home, allergic children often cannot help being exposed at school or during visits to relatives. Appropriate medicines given prior to exposure may help.

Mixed nuts are another problem. Even the odor causes trouble for some children. Others feel that they should avoid only peanuts, so they carefully select a different variety and then become ill because it has been in contact with peanuts.

Children allergic to eggs must be very careful not to drink eggnog at Christmas.

Holiday decorations can also precipitate allergies when brought out from storage in dusty and possibly musty or moldy areas. Some Christmas decorations used year after year (particularly stuffed ones) often have an "old" odor.

At Christmas time, in particular, children tend to become fatigued and overexcited. These factors can contribute to the onset of asthma.

### What Jewish holiday foods could cause allergies?

Although Jewish holidays such as Rosh Hashanah/Yom Kippur, Chanukah, Purim and Passover feature certain traditional foods, the majority of these dishes are also eaten throughout the year. Gefilte fish, eggs, spices, nuts, chicken, *kreplach* (containing eggs, wheat and spices), spiced and pickled herring, tuna fish, *challah* (ritual bread containing yeast and eggs), *farfel* (eggs and flour) and potato pancakes (wheat, eggs and onions) are typical examples.

The traditional Purim *hamantashen* (made with eggs, flour and some cooking oil) are usually filled with prunes or poppy seed, both of which can cause allergic reactions in some children. Passover *matzoh* (composed mainly of wheat, though flavorings or egg may be added) and the nuts and apples (if unwashed) of a specific Passover ritual dish could cause allergies from having been exposed to insecticides.

Wine, an adjunct to many Jewish holiday menus, could also be an allergy problem. In addition, *lox* (smoked salmon) can precipitate fish allergy, and candle odors can trigger asthmatic reactions. It should be remembered that decorations used on various holidays have been stored away and could be dusty.

### What other special days might trigger allergic symptoms?

THANKSGIVING—Cranberries and squash usually don't cause allergies but could in some children. Chestnuts, spices, special ingredients in turkey dressing or wine could also cause symptoms.

MOTHER'S DAY—Certain types of flowers or chocolates could cause symptoms in the allergic child.

JULY 4TH—The odor of firecrackers could trigger asthma, coughing or hay fever symptoms. This can also be irritating to persons without allergies.

BIRTHDAY PARTIES—All the usual birthday foods such as an egg-white cake frosting, nut flavoring or special coloring in the cake or icing, ice cream, chocolate, cinnamon or glazed apples. Burning birthday candles can be another allergy hazard. The mere excitement of the occasion could cause almost any of the typical symptoms of allergy. Give asthma medicines the day before and on the birthday itself, if the excitement always triggers wheezing.

# CHAPTER 20

# Traveling with an allergic child

**What are the major problems when traveling with an allergic child?**

MEDICINES—Be certain that you are well supplied with all the usual nasal and asthma medicines your child uses. Carry all, even if your child has not wheezed in years, because this may be just the time the problem reappears. If your child has sudden allergies or infection, take him to the nearest hospital or physician or call the county medical society if you don't know where to go. Know the exact names of your medicines, so that the doctor will have as much information as possible. Start antibiotics, if they are indicated, as soon as possible if your child's infection is usually associated with asthma.

FOODS—Carry your own unless you are certain that you can buy foods which will not cause allergic difficulty in your child.

SLEEPING—Be sure that any place where you stop to sleep looks and smells clean and is not musty or smoky. Carry your child's own synthetic pillow, if possible, and even a barrier cloth cover for the mattress, being careful to cover it *entirely* on top, bottom and ends. Woolen blankets must be sandwiched in the middle of the bedding, so they are not pulled directly under the child's nose.

If possible, carry a small de-pollution unit and use it constantly (even when you are not in the room) while at a motel or hotel. Place it in the room where the child is to sleep.

Special problems often arise when visiting relatives or friends whose homes are dusty or who have pets. Allergic children often start to wheeze, but parents are reluctant to go to a motel or return home earlier than anticipated because someone might be offended. If the child remains in such a home, the medical problem often becomes progressively more severe. One solution is to avoid difficulty entirely by staying at a motel if you anticipate that sleeping at someone's home may cause your child to become ill.

Don't smoke in a car while traveling. Cigarette or cigar smoke can aggravate or cause asthma, nasal and eye allergies. Don't burn insect-repellent or other candles or use cookers which cause irritating odors. The odor of chemical solutions used to ignite charcoal can precipitate symptoms.

MISCELLANEOUS FACTORS—Avoid fatigue and chilling. Don't travel to areas with high pollen counts when pollens are a problem (see pp. 278–281).

### How do you keep an extract refrigerated while traveling?

Put it in a thermos of ice. Change the ice whenever possible. Protect the extract label by wrapping it in a plastic bag and tying it very securely.

### Does freezing damage an extract?

Not usually, but it may cause a precipitate or clouding of a previously clear extract. This is true for aqueous (water) extracts rather than the longer-acting types (*e.g.*, Allpyral). The latter are normally cloudy and should never be frozen.

### Will it hurt the extract if it is kept at room temperature for a few days?

No. If the extract is sterile, it can be kept at room temperature for three to four days; to be safe, however, try to maintain the thermos-refrigeration.

### Where can your child receive an extract treatment when the family is traveling?

A hospital physician, or any other doctor who is willing to give it, can provide the treatment necessary.

### Will all physicians give the treatment?

No. Most would justifiably refuse to give an extract treatment if you do not have the following:

1. A well labeled extract bearing the child's name and a description of the contents. For example, "weed extract." The label must state the strength and should have an expiration date (e.d.).

2. Explicit instructions from your regular physician or allergist stating the exact dose, the name and strength of the extract and the date by which it should be given. If *any* of this information is lacking, the extract cannot safely be given.

When you obtain an extract and instructions from your regular doctor, be certain that you have *all* the above information clearly written out for you. Depend only on yourself for this, because the longer an extract dosage is overdue, the more problems your child may have when the extract is finally given. Example of labels:

| | |
|---|---|
| Tom Jones | Tom Jones |
| Grass Extract | Winter Extract |
| 10,000 p.n.u. | 1:100 |
| dose due by 12/30/79 | dose due by 12/30/79 |
| 0.6 cc 10,000 p.n.u. | 0.9 cc 1:100 |
| e.d. 1/30/80 | e.d. 1/30/80 |

**What common problem arises when allergy-extract treatments are given by someone other than your regular physician?**

When a child receives an allergy-extract treatment while traveling or at camp, it is not uncommon for him to return to his regular physician without any records of when or how much extract was given. If this situation might occur, be certain that the temporary replacement for your physician supplies this exact information. The date and dosage for your child's subsequent treatment are predicated upon this knowledge.

**What should you do about an allergy emergency when traveling?**

1. Phone your own allergist. The answer may be minutes away.

2. Take your regular allergy medications, *e.g.*, antihistamines and/ or asthma medicines. If unsure, take both.

3. Take Alka-Seltzer Antacid Formula (without aspirin) if a food conceivably could be causing the problem. If you have none, try one teaspoon of baking soda in a large glass of water.

4. Try to separate yourself from the offending item or exposure, if you know what is causing symptoms.

5. Go to the nearest hospital emergency room or physician. Oxygen and intravenous sodium bicarbonate sometimes relieve chemical- or food-sensitivity reactions in a few minutes.

**What tips might be helpful for college students?**

1. Take your own cotton pillow, cotton barrier cloth mattress and box spring covers. If you plan to room with someone, consider giving him similar covers. Your blankets should be washable cotton or wool, not odorous synthetics.

2. If you have an air-cleaner, use it either in the daytime or at night. This will help to eliminate dust.

3. Try to room with someone who also has allergies. Be certain you do not room with anyone who smokes or uses scented cosmetic preparations.

4. Take your books concerning how to cope with allergies. If problems arise, refer to them and if the answers aren't there, call your regular allergist or physician.

5. When having extract-treatments while at college, pay attention to the exact dosage and color of any extract which you normally receive. Each time you receive a treatment, watch to see if the amount and color seem correct. If not, speak up. If questions arise, urge that your own allergist be contacted *before* you receive your treatment. If you feel ill at ease at the college health center, take your extract to a local physician and receive your treatments there.

6. College students often have problems related to their allergy-extract treatments because of tight schedules near examinations and holidays. Anticipate such problems and receive your allergy treatment *earlier* than needed, so that you have one less pressure at these critical times.

7. If you return home and need your allergy treatment, it cannot be given safely if you do not have both the medicine and the record of the exact date and dosage of the last injection at school, *e.g.*, "0.7 ml 1:100 received 11/15, due for next treatment by 12/19." You must anticipate your needs *before* the college health service closes.

8. Keep your extract refrigerated.

9. For possible food sensitivities always keep Alka-Seltzer, *in gold foil,* in your wallet and room. If you have sudden allergic symptoms in any area of your body and are unsure of the cause, try this preparation. If a food is the cause of your medical problem, you may be fine in 20 minutes. If you have no Alka-Seltzer Gold, use baking soda, one teaspoon in one glass of water.

10. Take a little medicine kit with you to school. Include an aspirin substitute such as Tylenol or Tempra, Vitamin C (500 or 1000 mg tablets), an antihistamine, some nose drops and your asthma medicine. Take asthma medicines even if you have never wheezed.

# PART SEVEN

# Special aids to help those with allergies

THIS section helps patients determine where to purchase various items which have been recommended herein.

It explains unsuspected items which contain common allergenic food.

It gives various food aids to help those with major food allergies.

It lists common medicines by name to identify which allergic symptom a drug should relieve.

It has a pollen calendar for the United States to help you decide where and when you might take a vacation without exposure to a pollen to which you are sensitive.

# APPENDIX I

# Possible sources of known allergenic substances

## BUCKWHEAT

pancake flours or *kasha*
buckwheat grits, or cereal, is often used to line pans used to bake rye or
  pumpernickel bread. It prevents burning.

## CORN[1]

### SMELL

popping corn                     certain bath powders
boiling corn on cob              ironing certain starched clothes
certain body powders

### TASTE

corn flakes              grits
corn flour               hominy
corn meal                popped corn
corn oil (Mazola)        fresh corn
cornstarch               canned and frozen corn
corn sugars              succotash
corn syrups (Karo)

[1] From Theron G. Randolph, *Human Ecology and Susceptibility to the Chemical Environment,* 1972, Charles C. Thomas, Publisher, Springfield, Illinois. Used by permission.

## CORN IN SOME FORM

adhesives: envelopes, stickers, stamps, tapes
aspirin
bacon
baking mixes
baking powders[1]
beverages
bologna
breads or pastries
candy
catsup
Cheerios
chili
chop suey
coffee (instant)
confectioner's sugar
custards
dates
deep-fat frying oils
diluents for gelatin capsules, lozenges, ointments, suppositories, tablets
flour, bleached
fried foods
Fritos
frostings
fruit juices, especially grape juice
fruits
graham crackers
gravies
ham
jams
jellies
liquor (bourbon)
milk in paper cartons
monosodium glutamate
oleomargarine
pablum
paper containers (when wet)
peanut butter
pies, creamed
plastic food wrappers
Post Toasties
powdered sugar
puddings
salad dressing
salt
sandwich spreads
sauces for gravy, fish, meats, sundaes
sausages
sherbets
Similac
soups
soy-bean milks
teas (instant)
toothpastes or powders
tortillas
vegetables, especially beets, canned peas and string beans
vinegar
vitamins
wieners
yeasts
Zest

## COTTONSEED

candy, especially chocolate
cosmetics
cotton linters in furniture
cottonseed oil (Cooking oils, *e.g.,* Wesson, are believed to be nonallergenic.)
doughnuts
feed for cattle or poultry
fertilizer
fish
mayonnaise
miner's lamp oil

---

[1] See p. 303 for corn-free type.

oleomargarines such as Nucoa,
   Good Luck
potato chips
salad dressing

sardines may be in cottonseed oil
shortenings such as Crisco
some medicines such as
   camphorated oil

## FLAXSEED SOURCES

These include chair mats, cough remedies, depilatories, dust from linoleum, feed for animals, fiber board, flaxseed tea, insulating material, linen cloth, linseed-oil paints and varnishes, painters' and lithographic inks, plaster, Roman meal bread, straw hats, stuffing for furniture, wave-set lotions, wet printer's ink (boys with this sensitivity should not b newsboys or should wear gloves when delivering papers)

## GINGER

ginger ale, ginger beer, preserves, cookies or cake

## GUMS (VEGETABLE)

Indian, Karaya or Tragacanth are binders used to hold together tablet forms of medicine or to thicken foods or liquids, such as:

cake icing (commercially prepared)
cheeses (cream and others)
chewing gum
diabetic foods
denture adhesives
emulsified mineral oils
face powders
gelatins
gumdrop candy or jelly beans
ice-cream fillers
laxatives
lotions (hand and face)
lozenges

marshmallows
mouthwash
mustard
pie fillings
potato salad
rouge
salad dressing
soft-centered candy
toothpastes or powders
wave-set lotion
wheat cakes or flour
whipped cream
white sauces

## HAIR

### COW HAIR

blankets
brushes
certain carpets
"Ozite" rug pads (waffle-iron
   weave)
plaster

roofing felt for covering boilers or
   for insulation
rope
sofas and some cushions
stables or cows

## GOAT HAIR

artificial furs
blankets
carpets
cashmere clothing
felt hats
goats

mohair items—sweaters, suits, coats
mops
oriental rugs
plaster
ropes
water-proofing fabrics

## HOG HAIR

brushes
hogs
pads for rugs

## HORSEHAIR

certain hats
clothing exposed to horsehair
cushions
plasters
ropes

stables and horses
some brushes
some chairs
some mattresses
wigs

## RABBIT FUR OR HAIR

angora
coat trimming, muffs, rabbits'
   feet
felt hats

felt in sounding hammers of pianos
pillows, quilts, sweaters
rabbits or rabbit hutches

## ORRIS ROOT

This is a pulverized root used because of its faint, pleasant aroma. It may be found in bath salts, face powder or cream, hair tonic, lipstick, perfume, rouge, sachet powder, shampoo, shaving cream, scented soap, toothpaste and tooth powder.

Although many allergic patients are told to avoid pleasant-smelling substances because they can cause symptoms, most of these do not contain orris root. Scented substances which do not contain orris root may contain a volatile oil or some unknown substance which creates allergic symptoms. Something in scented facial and toilet tissue seems to cause allergies in some children, but it is not orris root.

## NON-ALLERGENIC COSMETICS

These can usually be purchased in large drugstores or department stores and should be tried if regular cosmetics cause allergies. Some brands are:

Allercreme
   Texas Pharmacal Company
      (Warner-Chilcott)
   307 E. Josephine
   San Antonio, Texas 78215

Ar-Ex Products
   1036 West Van Buren St.
   Chicago, Ill. 60607

Almay (Schieffelin and Co.)
850 Third Avenue
New York, N.Y. 10022

Do not use scented products.

# PYRETHRUM

Patients allergic to this substance frequently are also sensitive to ragweed or to plants in the chrysanthemum family because of a close botanical relationship. Florists or children frequently exposed to many flowers often become allergic to it. Pyrethrum is also found in some insecticides (both spray or powder), some plant sprays and some ointments or medicines used to treat skin parasites.

Children who have symptoms when exposed to insect sprays can sometimes tolerate a liquid (such as OFF) applied directly to the clothing. Never use sprays or chemicals if you have chemical allergies.

# KAPOK

This is a fiber of the silk-cotton tree found in Asia. It is silky and white and resembles dried milkweed-pod filling. It is used mainly to stuff toys, pillows, mattresses and comforters, and in upholstery and life jackets.

# SOYBEAN PRODUCTS (both meal and oil)[1]
(See soy-free diet pages, pages 317–323.)

## FOOD PRODUCTS

baked goods
candy, caramels, hard candy, nut candy
certain cereals, grits
certain diet foods
Chinese foods with soy sprouts
cooking oils
Crisco or Spry
ice cream
LaChoy sauce
lecithin, sometimes derived from soybean
margarine
mayonnaise
medicinal oil
milk substitutes as Sobee, Neo-Mull-Soy, Soyalac
pork sausage, wieners, lunch meats
seasoning powders
soups
soy nuts
wine (or in brewing of beer)
Worcestershire sauce

## INDUSTRIAL USES

Factories utilizing soy products can contaminate the air with enough of this substance to cause allergies in some very sensitive persons.

animal food
artificial wool
insecticides
leather dressing

[1] From Joseph H. Fries, Studies on the Allergenicity of Soybean, *Annals of Allergy,* 29:1, January, 1971. Used by permission of the author and publisher.

calking compound
candles
celluloid
cosmetics
disinfectants
electrical insulation
emulsifier
enamels
fertilizer
fire-fighting foam
fuel
glue and adhesives
glycerin

lighting
linoleum
oil cloth
paints
painting inks
plastics
rubber substitutes
soaps
synthetic resins
textile dressing
varnishes
waterpfoofing
whipping powder

# Food and diet aids

## COMMON RELATED FOODS AND GRAINS

If your child has obvious symptoms from one food in a group, it is possible the others might also cause difficulty.

apple, pear, quince
banana (plantain)
filbert, hazelnut, wintergreen
buckwheat, rhubarb
cashew, pistachio, mango
grapefruit, kumquat, lemon, lime, orange, tangerine
chocolate, cola
mushroom, yeast
beets, spinach, and lamb's quarters weed
cantaloupe, cucumber, pumpkin, squash, gherkin, melon
corn, barley, oats, rice, rye, wheat, sugar cane
blueberry, cranberry, huckleberry
avocado, bay leaf, cinnamon, sassafras
asparagus, chive, garlic, leek, onion, sarsaparilla, shallot
marshmallow, okra, cottonseed
lavender, oregano, peppermint, spearmint, sage, savory, thyme
broccoli, brussels sprouts, cabbage, mustard, radish, turnip, collards, cress,
    horseradish
allspice, clove
green or red pepper (cayenne), paprika, eggplant, white potato, tomato,
    coconut, date
anise, caraway seed, carrot, celery, dill, fennel, parsley, parsnip,
    acacia, lentils, peas, chick peas, beans (kidney, navy, pinto, string),
    licorice, soybeans, peanuts
almond, apricot, cherry, peach, plum
raspberry, blackberry, boysenberry, strawberry, loganberry
artichoke, burdock, chicory, dandelion, endive, lettuce, tarragon
black walnut, butternut, English walnut, hickory nut, pecan

## FISH FOODS

mollusks: clams, oysters, scallops
crustaceans: crabs, shrimp, lobster, crayfish

Since the following fish are in separate families, sensitivity to one may not indicate sensitivity to the rest.

    tuna
    whitefish
    white perch, yellow bass
    flounder, halibut
    grouper, sea bass
    cod, haddock
    anchovy
    pompano
    sardine, sea herring
    ocean perch
    marlin, sailfish
    salmon, trout
    caviar (sturgeon)
    picherd, pike
    yellow perch

If your child is sensitive to fish, he should avoid using Lepage's glue, or taking cod-liver oil tablets or liquid (see page 137). Fish glue is also found in book bindings and is used in furniture manufacture, rug sizing, shipping tapes and straw hats (see p. 130).

## POSSIBLE COMMON FOOD SOURCES OF
## MILK, WHEAT AND EGGS

| *Milk*[a] | *Wheat* | *Eggs* |
|---|---|---|
| au gratin foods | baked goods | albumin |
| baked goods[b,c] | biscuits | baked goods[f] |
| butter | breads[e,f] (including | Bavarian cream |
| candy[b] | rye, rice, etc.) | bread crumbs |
| casein or caseinate | bread crumbs | (at times) |
| cheese | breakfast cereals[b] | candy[b] |
| chocolate | candy[b] | coffee[b] |
| creamed or scalloped | coffee substitutes[b] | creamed foods |
| foods | crackers | croquettes |
| curds | cracker meal | crusts—if shiny |
| gravy | dumplings | (bread, etc.) |
| ice cream | gravy | custards |
| malted milk | macaroni, etc. | egg white or |
| margarine[d] | malt (beer) | powdered or |
| milk sherbet | noodles-spaghetti | dried egg |
| pudding | salad dressing | French ice cream |
| salad dressing | sauces for vegetable or | French toast |
| soups[b] | meat | fritters |
| waffle and biscuit | soups (bisques or | frostings |
| mixes | chowders) | meringue |
| whey | stuffing | noodles |
| white sauces | Swiss steak | pie filling |
| wieners or bologna[b] | wieners or bologna | root beer[b] |
| | | salad dressing |
| | | sauces |
| | | (Hollandaise) |
| | | sausage |
| | | soups[b] |

Note: Read all food labels very carefully.

[a] Kosher foods that contain neither milk nor meat are labeled "parve" and should not contain caseinate.

[b] Some, not all.

[c] Italian bread is *often* milk-free.

[d] Kosher margarine is acceptable.

[e] Make unseasoned Rykrisp sandwiches; all bread contains wheat.

[f] When baking, substitute ½ teaspoon baking powder for each egg omitted from the recipe.

Thanks are due to Dr. Jerome Glaser, of Rochester, N.Y., for much of the information in this list.

## RELATIVE DEGREES OF ALLERGENICITY OF FOODS

| *Often cause allergies* | *Sometimes cause allergies* |
| --- | --- |
| berries | apples |
| buckwheat | bacon |
| chocolate (cola) | bananas |
| cinnamon | beef |
| coconut | celery |
| corn | citrus fruits |
| egg white | (after infancy) |
| fish—all types, including crab, | cherries |
| lobster and shrimp | chicken |
| food coloring | coffee |
| milk | cottonseed |
| mustard | garlic |
| nuts—oil and | lettuce |
| extracts | melons |
| orange or citrus | mushrooms |
| (during infancy) | onion |
| peanut butter[1] | plum |
| peas | potatoes (white) |
| pork | prunes |
| sugar | spices |
| tomato products | spinach |
| wheat | soy products |
| yeast | vitamins |

---

[1] If your child is allergic to peanuts, be careful not to buy fried foods, such as doughnuts, cooked in peanut oil.

# Common Food Additives*

## CLASS OR TYPE OF FOOD ADDITIVES

**Nutrient Supplements**
Thiamine (vitamin $B_1$)
Riboflavin (vitamin $B_2$)
Niacin (vitamin $B_3$)
Iron
Vitamin A
Vitamin D
Potassium iodide

**Nonnutritive Sweeteners**
Saccharin
Calcium and sodium cyclamates
  (cyclo hexyl sulfamates)

**Preservatives**
Antioxidants (for fatty products)
  BHA (butylated hydroxyanisole),
  BHT (butylated hydroxytoluene.)
  NDGA (nordihydroguaiaretic
    acid)
  Propyl gallate
  Mold or Rope Inhibitors or
    Antimycotic Agents
  Sodium and calcium propionate
  Sodium diacetate
  Lactic acid
  Sorbic acids
  Sodium and potassium sorbates
Fungicides
Sequestrants
  Sodium, calcium and potassium
  salts of citric
  Tartaric, metaphosphoric, and
  pyrophosphoric acids

**Other**
Benzoic acid
Sodium benzoate, sulfur dioxide

**Emulsifiers**
Lecithin
Mono and diglycerides
Propylene glycol alginate

**Stabilizers and Thickeners**
Pectins
Vegetable gums (carob bean,
  carrageenan, guar)
Gelatin
Agar agar

**Acids, Alkalies, Buffers,
  Neutralizing Agents**
Ammonium bicarbonate
Calcium carbonate
Potassium acid tartrate
Sodium aluminum phosphate
Tartaric acid

**Flavoring Agents**
Amyl acetate
Benzaldehyde
Ethyl butyrate
Methyl salicylate
Essential oils
Monosodium glutamate

**Bleaching Agents:
  Bread Improvers**
Benzoyl peroxide
Oxides of nitrogen
Chlorine dioxide
Nitrosyl chloride
Chlorine
Potassium bromate
Ammonium chloride
Calcium sulfate
Ammonium phosphates
Calcium phoshates

* This list is used with the kind permission of James O'Shea, M.D.

# APPENDIX III

# *MISCELLANEOUS*

## Commonly-Used Asthma Drugs

| Drugs with ephedrine and theophylline | Drugs which contain mainly theophylline | Drugs similar to ephedrine (Beta-adrenergic) |
|---|---|---|
| Amesec | Accurbron [j] | Alupent[h] |
| Bronkolixir [oc] | Asbron | Brethine[h] |
| Bronkotab [oc] | Aerolate Jr., Sr. | Bricanyl[j] |
| Dainite | Aquaphyllin [j] | Metaprel[h] |
| Ectasule Jr., Sr.[c,g] | Brondecon | |
| Isuprel | Elixocon [i] | |
| Lufyllin | Elixophyllin SR[h] | |
| Marax | Fleet's theophylline rectal | |
| Marax DF [j] | units | |
| Mudrane | Luasmin | |
| Quadrinal | Neothylline [h,j] | |
| Tedral [b] | Phyllocontin[c] | |
| Tedral SA[c] | Quibron [j] | |
| Verequad | Slo-Phyllin [h] | |
| | Slophyllin GG [j] | |
| | Somophyllin-T[i,j] | |
| | Theobid | |
| | Theoclear | |
| | Theodur [c,h] | |
| | Theokin | |
| | Theolair [h] | |
| | Theophyl tablet[h,k] and SR[c] | |
| | Theospan[h,j] | |

[a] This dries mucus and decreases swelling of nasal tissue.
[b] See page 255 because Tedral is licorice-flavored.
[c] Available in an 8-to-12-hour tablet or capsule form (Helpful at bedtime).
[d] This is available in an eight-to-12-hour liquid form.
[e] This tends to cause children to become sleepy.
[f] This tends to keep children awake.
[g] This contains no theophylline and lasts eight to 12 hours.
[h] Contains no dyes—tablets or capsules.
[i] Contains no dyes or sugar.
[oc] Available without a prescription.
[j] Contains no dyes—liquid.
[k] Only chewable theophylline product available.

## Commonly-used Hay Fever Drugs

| *Antihistamines* | *Antihistamines with decongestants[a]* |
|---|---|
| Actidil[c] | Actifed[e,h] |
| Benadryl[d] | Demazin[e,oc] |
| Chlortrimeton[b,oc] | Dimetapp[b] |
| Dimetane[b,c] | Ornade[b] |
| Disophrol | Rondec |
| Extendryl | Rynatan[b,g] |
| Fedahist[f] | Triaminic[oc] |
| Forhistal | |
| Hispril | |
| Histadyl | |
| Optimine[f] | |
| Phenergan[d] | |
| Polarmine[b,c] | |
| Pyribenzamine[b,d] | |
| Ryna[oc,h] | |
| Tacaryl[b,e,h] | |
| Tavist[f] | |
| Teldrin[b] | |

[a] This dries mucus and decreases swelling of nasal tissue.
[b] Available in an eight-to-12-hour tablet or capsule form (helpful at bedtime).
[c] This is available in an eight-to-12-hour liquid form.
[d] This tends to cause children to become sleepy.
[e] This tends to keep children awake.
[f] Contains no dyes—tablets or capsules.
[g] Contains no dyes or sugar.
[oc] Available without a prescription.
[h] Contains no dyes—liquid.

# ODORS WHICH CAN TRIGGER ALLERGIC SYMPTOMS[1]

adhesive tape
aerosols
alcohol (rubbing)
ammonia
banana oil
bleaches, chlorine type
bubble bath or oils
buckwheat flour
burning wood, pine cones, candles, paper, trash
camphor
castor beans (flour or oil)
Christmas trees or decorations
cleaning fluid for clothing or windows
coal, gasoline, kerosene, oil, wood
cosmetics
cooking, especially fish or eggs or flour dust
creosote
chlorinated water
deodorants
detergents
disinfectants
dyes for cloth, cosmetics, or shoes
exterminating compounds
floor wax
frying foods
fumes from exhaust, garage, garbage or factory
gas from leaky stove or refrigerator

grease
hair preparations
incense
ink, marking pens
insect repellents (spray or candles)
insulation
moth balls
paints, paint thinners, varnish, lacquer, shellac
paper (news, ditto, carbon, mimeograph)
perfumes
plastic containers, cements
polish for fingernails, metal, shoe or furniture
polyurethane
phenol products (Lysol)
rubber bedding, paints or items
sanding or woodwork
scented facial and toilet tissues
smoke from any source, including cigarettes
soaps
sulfur dioxide
tar fumes, or tar-based shampoos and ointments
tobacco
turpentine
typewriter-ribbons or stencils
vegetables while cooking such as onions, peas, beans, cabbage and potatoes
wood—cedar or pine

[1] From Theron G. Randolph, *Human Ecology and Susceptibility to the Chemical Environment*, 1972, Charles C. Thomas, Publisher, Springfield, Illinois. Used by permission.

# UNUSUAL ITEMS WHICH MAY BE RESPONSIBLE
## FOR ALLERGIC SYMPTOMS[1]

air-conditioning
antibiotics, hormones, or preservatives in or on foods
artificial food colorings
artificial sweeteners
braces for teeth
clothes starch
cornstarch
cosmetics
dyes in medicines
fillings in teeth
mouthwash
nylon in any form
hair dyes and permanents
plastics in any form (plastic homemade toys)
rayon or cellulose clothing
shoe polish
toothpastes
Vaseline and petroleum products
water (softened, chlorinated, fluoridated)
waxes on fruits and vegetables

[1] From Theron G. Randolph, *Human Ecology and Susceptibility to the Chemical Environment*, 1972, Charles C. Thomas, Publisher, Springfield, Illinois. Used by permission.

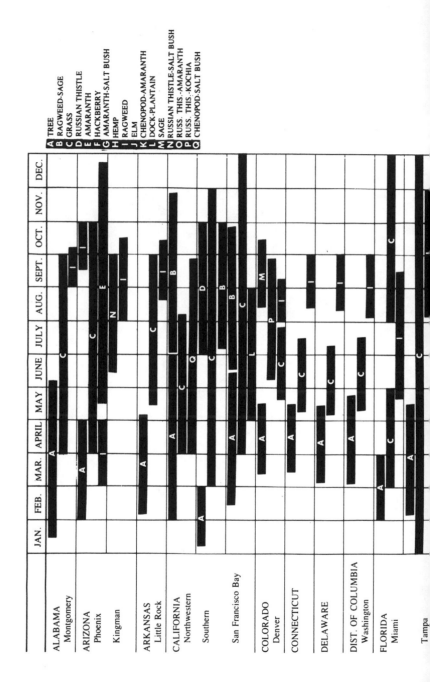

A TREE
B RAGWEED-SAGE
C GRASS
D RUSSIAN THISTLE
E AMARANTH
F HACKBERRY
G AMARANTH-SALT BUSH
H HEMP
I RAGWEED
J ELM
K CHENOPOD-AMARANTH
L DOCK-PLANTAIN
M SAGE
N RUSSIAN THISTLE-SALT BUSH
O RUSS. THIS.-AMARANTH
P RUSS. THIS.-KOCHIA
Q CHENOPOD-SALT BUSH

Pollen calendar from J. M. Sheldon, R. G. Lovell, K. P. Matthews, *A Manual of Clinical Allergy*, 2nd ed., 1967, W. B. Saunders, pp. 342–343. Used by permission.

Southern

ILLINOIS
Chicago

INDIANA
Indianapolis

IOWA
Ames

KANSAS
Wichita

KENTUCKY
Louisville

LOUISIANA
New Orleans

MAINE

MARYLAND
Baltimore

MASSACHUSETTS
Boston

MICHIGAN
Detroit

MINNESOTA
Minneapolis

MISSISSIPPI
Vicksburg

MISSOURI
St. Louis
Kansas City

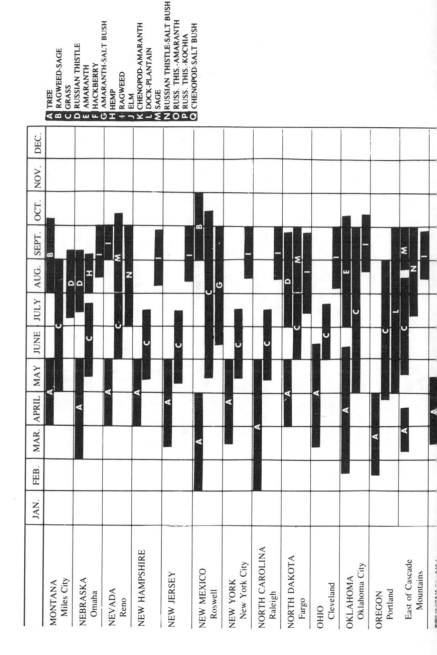

SOUTH CAROLINA
Charleston

SOUTH DAKOTA

TENNESSEE
Nashville

TEXAS
Dallas

Brownsville

UTAH
Salt Lake City

VERMONT

VIRGINIA
Richmond

WASHINGTON
Seattle

Eastern

WEST VIRGINIA

WISCONSIN
Madison

WYOMING

# Some sources of supplies and aids

The following are sources of products which may be useful to parents. The list is by no means complete and offers only possibilities, not specific endorsements.

For general information, write to the Asthma and Allergy Foundation of America, 19 West 44th St., New York, NY 10036.

## BEDROOM

*Cotton Products*

For 100-percent cotton fabrics, blankets, sheets, towels, washcloths, etc., write:

Ecologist's Co-op
2986 Talisman Drive
Dallas, TX 75229

Clothing and yarn are also available from the above.

Barrier cloth mattress covers which are unusually tightly woven are available in different sizes.

For natural cotton mattresses suitable for chemical-sensitive persons, write:

Scope Natural Fibers
1202 Carthage Rd.
Lumberton, NC 28358

For other information regarding cotton, write:

National Cotton Council of America
1030 15th St., N. W.—Suite 700
Washington, DC 20005

or

National Cotton Council of America
P. O. Box 12285
Memphis, TN 38112

# KITCHEN

*Cooking Aids*
Booklets:

*Baking For People With Food Allergies*
(Home and Garden Bulletin No. 147)
Supt. of Documents
U. S. Printing Office
Washington, DC 20402

The following booklets contain wheat, milk and egg-free recipes:

*Allergy Recipes*
The American Dietetic Association
620 North Michigan Ave.
Chicago, IL 60611

*Allergy Recipes From The Blue Flame Kitchen*
Metropolitan Utilities District
1723 Harney St.
Omaha, NE 68102

*125 Great Recipes For Allergy Diets*
Good Housekeeping Bulletin Service
959 8th Ave.
New York, NY 10019

For information about sugarless canned fruits, candies, cookies and gum, and individual flours (barley, oat, potato, rice, rye, corn, tapioca, etc.), rye bread, wheat-free cake, rice-cake and starch products, write:

Chicago Dietetic Supply Co.
P. O. Box 40
La Grange, IL 60525

Information is also available from:

The Rice Council of America
P. O. Box 22802
3917 Richmond Ave.
Houston, TX 77027

*Books:*

The following books may prove helpful:

*The Milk-Free & Milk-Free, Egg-Free Cook Book*
Isobel S. Sainsbury, M. D.
Charles C. Thomas, Publisher
301 East Lawrence Ave.
Springfield, IL 62717

*The Allergy Cook Book*
Carol G. Emerling and Eugene O. Johnson
Doubleday and Company, Inc., Publisher
Garden City, NY 11530

For *many* tips about cooking, foods and home:

*Coping With Your Allergies*
Natalie Golos and Frances Golbitz
Simon and Schuster, Publisher
1230 Ave. of the Americas
New York, NY 10020

*Allergy Cooking*
Marion L. Conrad
Pyramid Books, Publisher
919 Third Ave.
New York, NY 10022

*Oats, Peas, Beans, Barley*
Edyth Cottrell
Woodridge Press, Publisher
Santa Barbara, CA 93111

*Sugar Blues*
William Duffy
Warner Books, Publisher
75 Rockefeller Plaza
New York, NY 10019

*Natural Snacks 'N' Sweets*
Stan and Floss Dworkin
Rodale Press, Publisher
Emmaus, PA 18049

*Natural Cooking: The Prevention Way*
Charles Gerras, Ed.
Rodale Press, Publisher
Emmaus, PA 18049

*Resource Handbook on Allergies*
Kay Ludeman and Louis Henderson
Human Ecology Research Foundation
720 No. Michigan Ave.
Chicago, IL 60611

*Cooking For Your Hyperactive Child*
June Roth
Contemporary Publishers
180 North Michigan Ave.
Chicago, IL 60601

*The Food Depression Connection*
June Roth
Contemporary Publishers
180 North Michigan Ave.
Chicago, IL 60601
For additional books concerning cooking, see starred items on pp. 328–329.

# MISCELLANEOUS AIDS

*Dust Masks*
These masks may be helpful when cleaning dusty areas, painting or even when cutting the grass. One type is the Dustfoe 66 Respirator Mask. This is a quality product and can be obtained by writing:
Mine Safety Appliance Co.
519 Niagara St.
Tonawanda, NY 14150

(Or you may find it at local outlets.)

*Exercises*
For the booklet *Breathing Control for Asthma and Emphysema,* write:
The Asthma Research Council
12 Pembridge Square
Palace Court
London, England W2 4EH

*Air Cleaners and Purifiers*
Air-Conditioning Engineers
c/o Mr. H. Reed Miner
P. O. Box 616
Decatur, IL 62525
Also supplies small, portable purification units for air travel.

*Electrostatic Precipitation Units*
For local distributors, check the Yellow Pages of your telephone directory under "Air-Conditioning." Both small-room units and larger ones are available. Some recommended brands are General Electric, Micronaire and Westinghouse.
Recommended brands of furnace units are Electroair, Honeywell, Trane and Triton.

*Dehumidification Units*
Several suggested dehumidifiers are Comfort Air, Fedders, Oasis and Kelvinator. For more information, write:

ters Servicenter
ejoy St.
NY 14223

For chemically-sensitive persons, these units can be ordered stripped of all rubber and plastic parts.

*Name Tags*

Name tags must be worn by children who have drug, stinging-insect or severe food allergies. Older children might prefer to carry a card in their wallets stating the substance to which they are allergic. Be certain to buy only stainless steel tags because others may "turn green." These tags may be obtained from:

Medic Alert Foundation
P. O. Box 1009
Turlock, CA 95380

or

National Identification Co.
3955 Oneida St.
Denver, CO 80207

Neck chains are frequently lost, especially when boys swim, so bracelets are better. An attractive band for boys or girls is the Speidel Medical Alert Bracelet (silver). Links can be added as needed. Girls may prefer a gold heart pendant which can be engraved stating their name and type of allergy.

*Diminishing or Preventing Mold Allergy*

In order to diminish mold contamination in your home, you should:

—Remove all obviously moldy items, *e.g.,* carpets, luggage, shoes, wallpaper, books and plants.

—Wash items or parts which appear moldy but cannot be discarded, *i.e.,* humidifiers, air-conditioners, rubber refrigerator gaskets, room vaporizers, bathroom and shower tiles, window sills, etc. For cleaning (to protect against bacteria, molds or fungi) use Aqueous Zephiran (obtainable at drugstores) in a 17 per cent concentration. (Dilute as directed—one oz. concentrate per gallon of water or one tablespoon of concentrate per 27 tablespoons of water.) Be careful that it does not damage lightly varnished or finished furniture.

For captan (an agricultural fungicide obtainable from a tree nursery or garden-supply store) solutions, use four oz. of powder per gallon of water. Vinegar and water also may be used especially to reduce black mildew on refrigerator doors. Borax is a good mold-retardant. One can also use quatrammonium sulphate solution or the type used in swimming pools to control algae.

—Install a dehumidifier in basement or moldy area. (Heat, light and better circulation diminish mold growth.)

To prevent a mold allergy:

—Purchase a dry home situated on an elevated land area. Avoid homes which need sump pumps or have basements with water-level marks on the walls indicating previous flooding.

—Avoid bathroom walls steaming from frequent hot showers. Dry damp bathroom areas after showers.

—Avoid excessive use of vaporizers in bedroom.

—Cross-ventilate and heat basement or cellar. Seal basement wall cracks with silicone-rubber seal. (Odor of seal may cause symptoms in some patients.)

—Avoid large numbers of house plants, terrariums and home greenhouse units.

—Urge home builders to put sheets of heavy, black polyethylene under basement foundation and outside foundation wall to prevent leakage and mold problems.

—Don't rake wet leaves.

—Never leave damp clothes in washing machines or closets.

### Stinging-Insect Kit

This is available from Hollister-Stier Division, Cutter Laboratories, Inc., Yeadon, PA 19050. Most drugstores stock these during the summer months.

### Vacuum Cleaners

The best variety is a centralized vacuum with ducts leading into the basement. Next best is the portable water-tank type made by Rainbow Rexair. For information on this product, write:

Allied Vaccum Cleaner Co.
3110 Delaware Ave.
Buffalo, NY 14223

### Allergy-Free Vitamins

The following are firms that sell vitamins without food coloring, sugar or corn:

Willner Chemists
330 Lexington Ave.
New York, NY 10016

Vital Life
P. O. Box 618
Carlsbad, CA 92008

Carlson Natural Supplements
Feel Rite Health Food Store
1451 Hertel Ave.
Buffalo, NY 14216

Bronson Pharmaceuticals
4526 Rinetti Lane
La Canada, CA 91011

(Check at local health food stores for other brands.)

*Ecologists in the United States*

Physicians practicing ecology are both interested and trained in the diagnosis and therapy of health problems which appear related to foods, chemicals and various types of environmental contamination or pollution. They believe that susceptible individuals of all ages can have adverse reactions to natural and unnatural exposures in our food, water, air, drugs and homes. These doctors believe such exposure can cause maladaptation in afflicted persons, which can manifest in a wide variety of intermittent or constant, acute or chronic physical or mental symptoms. They stress avoidance and dietary manipulation, rather than drug therapy. Many treat patients using various forms of allergy-extract therapy if the patient does not respond to the above.

The Society for Clinical Ecology was founded in 1965 by a number of pioneers in this field, which included French Hansel, Herbert Rinkel, Jonathan Forman, Carlton Lee, Theron G. Randolph, George Frauenberger and Francis Silver. The growing membership includes a wide variety of medical and other specialists who recognize and appreciate the scope of this type of problem in our world. Names of physicians in your area who are also ecologists will be provided by:

Society For Clinical Ecology
Del Stigler, M.D., Secretary
2005 Franklin, Suite 490
Denver, CO 80205

Names of eye and ear specialists familiar with food testing and therapy will be provided by:

The American Society of Ophthalmologic and
    Otolaryngologic Allergy
William P. King, M. D., Secretary
1415 Third St.
Corpus Christi, TX 78404

The following is a list of physicians and hospitals which evaluate odd and unusual allergies through fasting and allergy environmental control:

Theron G. Randolph, M.D.
Hennrotin Hospital
111 West Oak St.
Chicago, IL 60610

(This unit is particularly interested in vascular problems and arthritis·¨

William Rea, M. D.
Carrollton Community Hospital
1711 South Broadway
Carrollton, TX 75006

Presbyterian Medical Center
1719 East 19th Ave.
Denver, CO 80218

Marshall Mandell, M. D.
The New England Foundation for
    Allergic and Environmental Diseases
3 Brush St.
Norwalk, CT 06850

(Particularly interested in arthritis evaluation:)

Francis Carroll, M. D.
722 North Brown St.
Chadbourn, NC 28431

# APPENDIX V

# *Bioassay Titration Skin Testing*

This new method of testing has been applied to help detect allergies to dust, pollens, mold spores, pets, foods, some chemicals, hormones, flu vaccines, stinging insects, antibiotics or other drugs. It is highly controversial at present, but a growing number of physicians are beginning to apply the basic principles of this type of practice after confirming their personal observations that this form of therapy is effective. Rigorous scientific studies are presently being designed to confirm or deny the efficacy of these newer methods. The final answers will not be known for several years.

The patient is tested with a number of dilutions (two to ten) for each specific allergy extract. If the dilution is too strong or too weak, the patient may have a flare of symptoms, a rise in pulse, a large local reaction to the skin test, or a fall in the breathing test (Peak Flow Meter) indicating asthma. When the "correct" dilution or range is found, the patient often notes that the symptoms subside, the pulse returns to normal, the local skin reaction is not unusual and the breathing test improves. All these changes do not occur in each patient with each test, but all are indices to help the physician determine the "correct" dosage to use for treatment.

Some physicians test by starting with weak dilutions and gradually use stronger concentrations, while others start with strong solutions and gradually test with progressively weaker dilutions. Some start with intermediate-strength dilutions and go weak or strong depending upon the patient's reactions. Some test the patients by using superficial skin tests, others use deeper skin tests and some do the testing under the tongue (sublingually). In general, the results appear to be similar, regardless of the type of expertise which a particular physician utilizes.

The RAST test (p. 185) appears to enable a physician to determine from the blood serum approximately the "correct" dilution to use for treating some patients who have an allergy to pollens, mold spores, dust, stinging insects and some foods. This can greatly reduce the need for allergy skin testing for these items. This test, unfortunately, is not presently helpful for the diagnosis or treatment of the majority of food or chemical sensitivities.

The patient is tested with a small or large number of potentially allergenic substances. The number varies from patient to patient depending upon the history given to the physician. For example, if the problem is present during a single pollen season, only that particular pollen might be tested. If the symptoms are year-round, and worse during the pollen seasons, the patient might need complete testing for allergenic items within and outside the home, as well as for foods. If the problem began early in infancy, food testing would be indicated.

Once testing is completed, the patient can be treated with a number of combinations of the various items tested. The "correct" dose of each item is placed into the treatment solution. For example, there may be one extract which contains food items and a second which contains dust, pollen, molds and pet dander. The treatment material can be administered by the patient sublingually with drops, or given by injection into the arm or leg by the physician or patient. The treatments may be needed one to three times a day at first but, as time passes, they gradually appear to be needed less and less often. The patient can tell when more treatment is needed because the symptoms recur. The patient's symptoms often subside within ten to 20 minutes after a treatment is taken. Patients who respond well to therapy often need to take little or no supplementary medication.

Unfortunately, patients with chemical allergy routinely cannot be treated for this problem. Avoidance is the most helpful form of therapy and this can be most challenging, difficult and expensive in our chemically contaminated, modern world.

The major disadvantage of this form of testing is that it is very time consuming. Suspect offending items may have to be checked individually until the "correct" treatment dose for each is found. Patients must be examined and watched carefully before and after each test. This raises the cost to the patient. Initially it increases the length of time and the number of visits to the physician.

The major advantage of this new therapy is that some patients appear to respond favorably within days to weeks. The need for drugs is markedly reduced, if not eliminated. Treatment often enables patients to eat in moderation the foods to which they are sensitive. The testing often can be self-administered, reducing visits to the physician's office. If an extract is no longer effective, it indicates a need for retesting which is fortunately required in only a relatively small number of patients. Successful therapy enables many patients to eat and live more normally.

Much more research is needed to rigorously study this form of therapy properly. In time we must learn the mechanism by which patients appear to be helped. It is surely not a panacea for the many illnesses which plague humanity but it appears to be a significant step in the right direction. The emphasis in medicine must change from treatment of the effect to elimination of the cause. The next challenge is to try to alter the body from within so that our basic homeostatic mechanisms can be restored, thus allowing normal living and eating, provided the body is not overwhelmed with too many environmental chemicals, toxins, industrial poisons or pollutants.

# Diets to check for various allergies

(The following pages have been adapted from the booklet *Food Sensitivity Diets*, © 1978 by Doris J. Rapp, and are used by permission of Syntex Laboratories.)

## DIET TO CHECK FOR MILK ALLERGY[1]

If you want to confirm the presence of a milk allergy, try the following:

First: Only "allowed" foods listed below are permitted for one or two full weeks. Notice if the patient is the same or better in any way when milk or milk-containing foods are not consumed.

Second: Check with your doctor after all milk products have been stopped for two weeks (or sooner if the patient is perfectly well). Your doctor will decide when these foods should be re-added to the diet. If symptoms recur, check with your doctor.

## ALLOWED

Beverages or drinks:
  Carbonated beverages such
    as pop
  Kool-Aid
  Coffee Rich
  Soybean-type milk, Soy-base
    formula

Juice from canned fruits
Margarines
  Use only:
  Diet Imperial
  Mother's

---

[1] Read baby food labels *very carefully*. Many baby foods contain milk. For soybean milk recipes, write for the free NEO-MULL-SOY® Formula Recipe Book published by Syntex Laboratories, Inc., Nutritional Products Division, 3401 Hillview Ave., Palo Alto, CA 94304.

Mrs. Filbert's Diet Spread
Safflower
Any Kosher *Parve* brand[1]
Fruits (any fresh type in any
form)
Vegetables (all allowed except
creamed types)
Cereals (all allowed if Coffee
Rich, fruit juice or soybean
milk is used on top of cereal
instead of milk)
Baked goods (any, providing
not made with butter or any
type of milk)
Breads:
   *Challah*
   Rye breads:
      Only the following:
      Grossman's
      Beefsteak
      Kaufman's
      Millbrook Swedish &
         Dixie Rye
      Arnold's Jewish Rye
   Italian breads:
      Only the following:
      Balisteri's
      Maria's
      Marzolina's
      Ontario
   (Brand names vary in
      different parts of the
      country—check with your
      doctor.)

Meats:
   All fresh meats
   Kosher luncheon meats, hot
      dogs, bologna and salami
      Sinai brand
      Hebrew National (may be
         very spicy)
      "393"—all-beef hot dogs
   All poultry without stuffing
All fish
Desserts and snacks (any,
   providing it is not made with
   butter or any type of milk):
   Some examples:
      Abel's Bagels
      Ritz Crackers
      Salerno Saltines
      Stella D'Oro Cookies
      Voortman's Apple
         Oatmeal Cookies
      Soy-base Ice Cream (see
         p. 174)
Miscellaneous:
   Hershey's Special Bar
   Cocoa: Hershey or Baker's
   Bitter Baking Chocolate
   Ontario Bread Crumbs
   Any kosher food labeled
      *Parve* or *Pareve*
   Milk of Magnesia
   CHO-free milk

---

[1] Kosher milk-free foods (*Parve* or *Pareve*) are available at any Jewish delicatessen, or the kosher food section in large supermarkets.

## NOT ALLOWED

Beverages or drinks:
- Milk (cow's or goat's)
- Skimmed milk
- 2% milk
- Buttermilk
- Whole milk
- Chocolate milk or drink
- Malted milk
- Coffee-mate
- Dry milk
- Evaporated milk
- Powdered milk
- Acidified milk

Milk Products
- Butter
- Casein or sodium caseinate
- Cheese
- Curds
- Ice cream
- Margarine (except those listed above)
- Whey
- Cottage Cheese
- Yogurt

Fruits (read labels on all fruit desserts)

Vegetables (any creamed type, *e.g.*, corn, peas, etc.)

Cereals:
- Country Morning
- Granola
- Baked goods (allow none if baked with butter or any type of milk. Allow no item with casein, sodium caseinate or whey in ingredients)

Breads (eat only those listed above):
- Arnold's
- Millbrook
- Profile
- Tops
- Wonder

Meats:
- Non-kosher luncheon meats
- Bologna
- Salami
- Wieners
- Sausage
- Meat loaf
- Cold cuts
- Meatballs

Desserts and snacks (allow none that contain butter, milk, casein, sodium caseinate, or whey, which may be found in many):
- Cookies
- Candy (especially cremes, chocolates, opaque candy)
- Chocolate (milk chocolate and some dark chocolate)
- Ice cream and milk sherbert
- Pudding
- Waffle and biscuit mixes

Crackers (most snack crackers)
- Saltines
- Sara Lynn store brand
- Sunshine

Miscellaneous
- Au gratin foods
- Creamed or scalloped foods
- Gourmet foods with cheese or milk
- Gravy
- Lactose
- Soups
- White sauces

## DIET TO CHECK FOR WHEAT ALLERGY

If you want to confirm the presence of a wheat allergy, try the following:

First: Only "allowed" foods listed below are permitted for one or two full weeks. Notice if the patient is the same or better in any way when wheat or wheat-containing foods are not consumed.

Second: Check with your doctor after all wheat products have been stopped for two weeks (or sooner if the patient is perfectly well). Your doctor will decide when these foods should be re-added to the diet. If symptoms recur, check with your doctor.

## ALLOWED

Cereals (any which do not
  contain wheat)
  Corn (corn flakes)
  Rice
    Rice Krispies
    Puffed Rice
  Oat
  Barley
  Soy
  Rye (grind up Rykrisp
    crackers)[1]
Beverages
  Milk (regular, skimmed, 2%)
  Fruit juice
  Soda pop
  Kool-Aid
  Soybean milk
  Buttermilk
  Chocolate drink (check label)
Fruits and vegetables (all fresh
  fruits and vegetables; canned
  and frozen fruits and
  vegetables if not creamed,
  stewed or otherwise prepared
  with wheat)
Baked goods (any which do not
  contain wheat)

Use flours other than wheat
  such as:
  Rice (muffins or bread)
  Barley
  Potato starch
  Oat
  Soya
    (READ LABELS
    CAREFULLY)
  All rye and potato breads
  usually contain wheat
  except:
    Bayern Schnitten
    Rye bread (Loblaw's)
Meats (all fresh meats, poultry,
  fish except those prepared
  with wheat)
Desserts and snacks (any which
  do not contain wheat—see
  Baked goods)
  Fruit ice or sherbet
Soups (any which do not
  contain wheat)
Miscellaneous

[1] Some patients with a wheat allergy may react to Rykrisp.

To make all-purpose flour
without wheat, mix:

1 cup cornstarch +

2 cups rice flour +

2 cups soya flour +

3 cups potato
starch flour

Use equal cups of this mixture
to replace wheat flour in
recipe for baking. Bake at
lower temperature for longer
period of time. Will be
crustier.

Flour exchange: 1 cup wheat
flour=

1⅛ cup rolled oats

or

1 cup rye meal

or

1¼ cups rye flour

or

¾ cup soya flour

or

⅝ cup potato starch flour

or

⅞ cup rice flour

or

½ cup barley flour

or

¾ cup cornmeal

Thickening exchange: 1
tablespoon wheat
flour=approximately ½
tablespoon cornstarch

or

½ tablespoon potato starch
flour

or

½ tablespoon arrowroot flour

or

2 teaspoons quick tapioca

## NOT ALLOWED

Cereals

   All which contain wheat, *e.g.*

      Cream of Wheat

      Farina

      Grapenuts

      Puffed Wheat

      Ralston's Shredded Wheat

      Triscuits

      Wheatena

      Cheerios

      Wheat germ

Beverages

   Postum

   Malted milk

   Ale

   Beer

   Wines (some)

   Gin

   Whiskies

   Coffee substitutes

   Ovaltine

Fruits and vegetables
  Stewed fruits
  Fruits contained in pies and jam
  Creamed vegetables
  Baked beans and chili con carne
Baked goods (most are forbidden)
  Bread and breadcrumbs
  Biscuits and biscuit mixes
  Cakes, cake mixes, cake flour
  Cookies
  Crackers and cracker meal
  Doughnuts and doughnut mixes
  Matzos
  Melba toast
  Pancake mixes
  Pies and pastry
  Popovers
  Potato flour
  Rusks
  Rye bread
  Waffles and waffle mixes
  Yeast (except zwieback)
Meats
  Breaded
  Canned
  Swiss steak
  Hot dogs and lunch meats
  Premolded hamburger
  Sausage
  Meat loaf
  Meatballs

Desserts and snacks
(see Baked Goods)
  Chocolate candy
  Cheese spreads and sauces
  Ice cream (including cones)
  Custard
  Puddings
  Sherbets
Soups
  (most soups:
    Campbell's Tomato Soup)
  Bouillon cubes
    Creamed soups
    Chowders
    Bisques
Miscellaneous
  Butter
  Cream sauce
  Dumplings
  Egg dishes
    (thickened with flour)
  Fritters
  Gravy
  Macaroni (noodles,
    ravioli, spaghetti)
  Salad dressings
  Scalloped dishes
  Wheat germ

For special school lunches, try:
  Homemade soups
  Fresh fruit
  Vegetable wedges and sticks
  Rykrisp sandwiches
  Chicken drumsticks (unbreaded)
  Pork chops (unbreaded)
  Potato chips (without additives or preservatives)
  Fresh fruit or vegetable salad

## DIET TO CHECK FOR EGG ALLERGY

If you want to confirm the presence of an egg allergy, try the following:

First: Only "allowed" foods listed below are permitted for one or two full weeks. Notice if the patient is the same or better in any way when eggs or egg-containing foods are not consumed.

Second: Check with your doctor after all egg products have been stopped for two weeks (or sooner if the patient is perfectly well). Your doctor will decide when these foods should be re-added to the diet. If symptoms recur, check with your doctor.

## ALLOWED

Egg Replacers (Jolly Joan brand)

Beverages (all except those listed in the NOT ALLOWED section below)

Fruits and vegetables (be careful of salad dressings containing eggs)

Baked goods (any which do not contain eggs in any form)

Jell-O pie filling (vanilla and lemon may be egg-free—read label)

Desserts and snacks (any which do not contain eggs)

Meats (all fresh meats, poultry, fish except those prepared with eggs such as those listed under Meats in the NOT ALLOWED section)

Miscellaneous

(When baking, substitute ½ tsp. egg-free baking powder for each egg omitted from the recipe. Buy this at a health store.)

To replace an egg in a recipe:

1. If a recipe calls for 2 tsp. baking powder and 2 eggs, merely use 3 tsp. egg-free baking powder or

2. Jolly Joan Egg Replacer (obtain at a health food store)
   1 tsp. Jolly Joan Egg Replacer + 3 tsp. water = 1 egg.
   For a recipe needing 2 eggs, use 2 tsp. Jolly Joan
   Egg Replacer plus 6 tsp. water.

## NOT ALLOWED

Eggs (in any form)

Albumin

Egg white (meringue) and yolk

Powdered or dried egg
Fleischmann's Egg Beaters or similar products

Beverages
Coffee or wine (if permitted)
Beverages containing eggs (read label)
Egg nog
Root beer (some brands)
Ovaltine (and Ovomalt)
Ovomucin, ovomucoid

Fruits and vegetables
None with Hollandaise sauce

Baked goods
Bavarian creams
Breads (especially those with shiny crusts)
Cakes
Cream pies
Doughnuts
Fritters
Meringue
Pancakes and waffles
Some pie fillings

Desserts and snacks
Candy (most)
Custards
French ice cream
Pretzels
Pudding

Meats
Fritter batter (fish)
Sausages
Egg dip used in breading liver, pork chops, chicken

Miscellaneous
Marshmallows
Bread crumbs (some)
Creamed foods
Croquettes
French toast
Fritters
Frosting
Ovetin
Noodles

Salad dressing
Sauces (Hollandaise or Tartar)
Soups (noodle, consommes)
Souffles
Spaghetti
Vitellin

## DIET TO CHECK FOR CHOCOLATE ALLERGY

To confirm the presence of a cocoa allergy, it is necessary to eliminate any food or drink containing chocolate for one to two weeks. When chocolate is then re-added to the diet, the patient should be encouraged to eat as much as possible to see if it affects the nose, ears, skin, chest, disposition, activity or causes bed-wetting. If chocolate in any form causes obvious symptoms, it must not be eaten before consulting your doctor.

### ALLOWED

Beverages
  Carob
  Cara Coa[1]
  Fruit juices or fruit beverages

Milk
Milk substitutes
  Isomil,® SoBee,® Nursoy,®
  Soyalac®

Substitutes for chocolate which look and taste like chocolate but contain none are available at large grocery stores or health food stores. Some do not have an acceptable taste.

Serve only the foods on the "Allowed" lists unless you already know the patient is allergic to one of them.

### NOT ALLOWED

Chocolate with colored (dyed)
  coating (brown, green, pink,
  yellow or white)
Chocolate in any:
  Drink
  Candy
  Baked goods

Cake
Cookies
Ice Cream
Any cola drinks
  Pepsi-Cola
  Coca-Cola
  Diet cola

[1] Information about Cara Coa chocolate substitute can be obtained from El Molino Mills, 345 North Baldwin Park Blvd., City of Industry, CA 91744.

Dr. Pepper
Miscellaneous
    Doritos Taco Chips (have
        cocoa)
    Vegetable gums (Karaya)

## DIET TO CHECK FOR CORN ALLERGY

If you want to confirm the presence of a corn allergy, try the following:

First: Only "allowed" foods listed below are permitted for one or two full weeks. Notice if the patient is the same or better in any way when corn or corn-containing foods are not consumed.

Second: Check with your doctor after all corn products have been stopped for two weeks (or sooner if the patient is perfectly well). Your doctor will decide when these foods should be re-added to the diet. If symptoms recur, check with your doctor.

## ALLOWED

Beverages
    Coffee (brewed)
    Dole Pineapple Juice
    Kool-Aid[1]
    Milk (in glass containers)
    Soy-base formula
    Orange juice (Minute Maid
        brand *only*)
    Tea (brewed)
    Tomato juice
    Welch's Grape Juice
    Bacardi Rum
    Michelob Beer (contains
        rice)
    14% Wine
    Milk (all milk if in glass or
        plastic containers)
Cottage cheese
Butter

Fruits (any fresh fruit)
Vegetables (any fresh
    vegetables)
Baked goods (homemade)
Cereals:
    Non-pre-sweetened types
        such as:
    Cream of Wheat
    Oatmeal
    Puffed Rice
    Rice Chex
    Rice Krispies
    Wheat Chex
    Wheaties
Bread (homemade with special
    ingredients—corn-free baking
    powders and yeast)
Meats (fresh meats)
    Beef

---

[1] Sweetened with honey.

Chicken
Pork
Veal

Sweeteners
  Beet sugar
  Honey
  Pure maple sugar
  Cane sugar
  Saccharin

Desserts and snacks
  Baker's chocolate
  Candy made with honey
  Cocoa
  Freshly-ground peanut butter
  Hershey's chocolate
  Maple candy (pure)
  Rykrisp

Baking ingredients
  Baking powder—Cellu (corn-
    free)

Ditex Baking Powder
Red Star Dry Yeast
Safflower oil
Tapioca
Unbleached flour
Wesson Oil

Medicines
  Actifed
  Cecon
  Cyrobeta
  Histadyl
  Hydryllin
  Upjohn's non-allergenic line
    of drugs
  Vitamin B
  Vitamin C
  Miscellaneous

Use Wesson Oil (cottonseed) or any type which is NOT corn
Use tapioca or flour instead of cornstarch for a thickening agent for
gravies.
TRY TO AVOID ALL OBVIOUS AND HIDDEN SOURCES OF
CORN. READ ALL LABELS!

## NOT ALLOWED

Beverages or drinks
  Most 7 Up
  Beer (except Michelob
    brand—contains rice)
  Ale
  Gin
  Vodka
  Whiskey
  Fortified wines and many
    liquors
  Canned or bottled juice
  drinks:
  Frozen orange juice (except

  Minute Maid)
  Hawaiian Punch
  Hi-C
  Mott's Apple Juice
  Some cranberry juice
  Coffee (instant)
  Coffee Rich

Infant formulas:
  Enfamil
  Evaporated milk
  SMA
  Similac

Fruits
  Candied fruits
  Canned fruits
  Dried fruits
  Frozen fruits (sweetened)
  Fruit desserts
Milk products
  Cheese (none except cottage
    cheese)
  Ice cream
  No milk in paper containers
Margarine
Sherbet
Yogurt
Vegetables
  Corn[1]
  Hominy[1]
  Succotash[1]
Baked goods
  All commercial baked
    goods
  Biscuits
  Bisquick
  Cake mixes
  Cookies
  Doughnuts
  Golden Mix
Pancake mixes
Pie crusts
Py-O-My
Cereals
  Alpha Bits
  Cheerios
  Corn flakes
  Pablum
  Post Toasties
  All pre-sweetened cereals
  Sugar-coated rice cereals
Breads (all commercial breads)

Meats
  Bacon
  Cooked meats in gravies
  Ham (cured)
  Luncheon meats (bologna,
    etc.)
  Sandwich spreads
  Sausages
  Wieners
Sweeteners
  Brown sugar
  Confectioners' sugar
  Corn sugars
  Corn syrup
  Pancake or waffle syrup
    (corn syrup, Karo syrup)
Desserts and snacks
  Candy
  Carob (Cara Coa chocolate)
  Cream pies
  Cookies
  Custard·
  Frostings
  Fritos
  Graham crackers
  Ice cream
  Jellies
  Jell-O
  Peanut butter
  Popcorn
  Pudding
  Sherbet
Baking ingredients
  All usual baking powders
    contain corn.[2]
  All corn oils (Mazola)
  All yeast (except Red Star
    Dry Yeast)
  Corn meal

[1] Not canned, creamed or frozen.
[2] Available at health food store—corn-free baking powder or yeast.

Cornstarch

Medicines
  Aspirin
  Bufferin
  Capsules
  Ointments
  Suppositories
  Vitamins
  Most medicines in tablet or
    pill form
  Disodium chromoglycate (Intal)

Miscellaneous
  No bath or body powders
  Cooking fumes of popcorn or
    fresh corn
  Paper cups and plates

Adhesives:
  Envelopes
  Labels
  Stickers
  Tapes
  Stamps
Liquids from paper cartons
Some plastic food wrappers
Toothpaste/powder
Foods fried in corn oil
Gravies
Monosodium glutamate
Zest Soap
Fructose, Dextrose
Sorbitol
Intravenous Dextrose

## CITRUS-FREE DIET

Some patients are allergic to citrus and others to citric acid. (See also p. 307—Citric Acid-Free Diet—to determine if the patient is allergic to either or both.)

## ALLOWED

Non-citrus fruits and juices:
Bottled juices
  Apple
  Grape (Welch's brand)
  Prune
  Cranberry
  Pear
  Peach
  Apricot
  Pineapple
  Tomato
Beverages
  Cola
  Cherry pop
  Root beer
  Vegetable juice

Miscellaneous
  Popsicles
  Grape
  Root beer
  Banana
Desserts
  Homemade jelly or jam
  made without citrus

## NOT ALLOWED

Citrus fruits and juices
    Orange
    Grapefruit
    Lemon
    Lime
    Kumquat
    Tangerine

Avoid any of the following, if flavoring is citrus:

Beverages
    Soda pop
        7 Up
        Squirt
        Teem
        Uptown
        Kool-Aid
        Hi-C
        Constant Comment Tea

Medicines
    Liquids
    Tablets
    Flavor-coated pills
    Lozenges
    Cough drops

Desserts
    Jell-O
    Candy and gum
    Sherbet
    Some jelly or jam

CHECK ALL LABELS CAREFULLY FOR FOODS CONTAINING CITRUS. IF IN DOUBT, CHECK WITH YOUR DOCTOR! If a food contains "citric acid," it may not necessarily contain citrus. However, some patients are allergic to *both* citric acid and citrus and must avoid both.

## CITRIC ACID-FREE DIET

### ALLOWED

Fruits and juices
- Apple[1]
- Banana
- Cherry[1]
- Grape[2]
- Cranberry
- Prune
- Pear[3]
- Peach[3]
- Apricot[3]

Beverages
- Cola

- Cherry pop
- Root beer (Shasta brand)
- Vegetable juice

Miscellaneous
- Popsicles
- Root beer
- Banana
- Some medicines, candy and cough drops
- Homemade jelly or jam without citric acid

Foods containing acids other than citric, *e.g.,* ascorbic acid (Vitamin C) are acceptable.

### NOT ALLOWED

Fruits and juices
- Orange
- Grapefruit
- Lemon
- Lime
- Pineapple
- Tomato
- Kumquat
- Tangerine

Beverages and desserts
- Jell-O
- Suckers
- Pop (7 Up, Squirt, Teem, Uptown)

- Sherbet
- Candy, gum
- Baked goods
- Pies
- Kool-Aid
- Hi-C

Medicines
- Liquids
- Alka-Seltzer (in Gold Foil)
- Vitamins
- Tablets
- Flavor-coated pills

[1] Bottled, not canned.

[2] Welch's juice in bottles.

[3] Available at health food store.

Lozenges
Cough drops
Snacks (*e.g.,* Munchos)
Store brands of jelly or jam
    made with citric acid

A beverage labeled "drink," such as "grape drink," means citric acid has been added.   CHECK ALL LABELS FOR CITRIC ACID-CONTAINING FOODS. IF IN DOUBT, CHECK WITH YOUR DOCTOR.


## DIET TO CHECK FOR SUGAR ALLERGY

If you want to confirm the presence of a sugar allergy, try the following;

First: Only the "allowed" foods listed below are permitted for a full seven to 14 days. Keep an exact record of everything eaten during this period of time. Notice if the patient is the same, better or worse in any way when sugar or sugar products are not consumed.

Second: Check with your doctor as soon as the patient is better, or on the fourteenth day if no improvement is noted. He may want sugar re-added to the diet. If so, notice if any symptoms occur within an hour. Symptoms may be helped by Alka-Seltzer (in gold foil). Remember, do *not* re-add sugar to the diet without the doctor's permission.


## ALLOWED

Sweeteners
    Honey
    Saccharin
    Real maple syrup or sugar
    Date sugar (obtainable at
    health food store)
Beverages
    Coffee (brewed, without
    sugar)
    Tea (brewed, without sugar)
    Natural fruit juice
    Mott's Apple Juice
    Dole Pineapple Juice
    Welch's Grape Juice

Tops Orange Juice
Minute Maid Orange Juice
Lincoln Apple Juice
Cereals
    Cream of wheat
    Cream of rice
    Oatmeal
    Puffed wheat (plain)
    Puffed rice (plain)
Baked goods (all homemade)
    Most Italian breads
    Most Italian rolls
    *Some* soda crackers (such as
        Premium Saltines)

Rykrisp
Fruits
  Fresh
  Frozen (without syrup)
Vegetables
  Frozen
  Blue Boy canned vegetables
  Fresh vegetables
Meats
  Fresh cut meats
  Plain smoked meats
  Poultry
Snacks
  Salted nuts
  Maple sugar candy
  Candy made with honey[1]
  Dates
  Raisins (unsulphured)
  Dried fruits without sugar
  Sesame candy bars (available
    at health food store)
  Potato chips (pure)
  Popsicles® made from sugar-
    free juice (homemade)

Toasted soy beans (available
  at health food store)
Rykrisp
Dairy products
  All milk—2%, skimmed,
    regular, non-fat
  Butter
  Sour cream
  Cottage cheese
  Yogurt (plain)
  Milkshakes made with fruit
    and honey
  Brick cheeses
Miscellaneous
  Most tablet medicines
  Mustard
  Oil & vinegar dressing
  Dietetic dressing
  Horseradish
  Homemade peanut butter
  Toothpowder made from salt
    and baking soda
  Eggs

Sugar can be made from cane, corn, beets, maple syrup or dates. Cane, corn or beet sugars cause allergy most frequently. A patient may be sensitive to only one type. READ ALL LABELS! INGREDIENTS MAY CHANGE!

## NOT ALLOWED

Sweeteners
  Sugar (granulated, powdered,
    brown, cane, beet)

Corn syrup
Store brand maple sugar

[1] Bake or make candy with honey instead of sugar. (1 cup honey = 1 cup sugar, but liquid must be reduced by ¼ cup. For example, for a recipe for 1 cup of sugar and 1 cup of milk, use 1 cup honey and ¾ cup milk.) Write to the following for further information: American Honey Institute, 831 Union Street, Shelbyville, Tennessee 37160; California Honey Advisory Board, P.O. Box 32, Whittier, California 90608.

Beverages
  Most rum
  Instant coffee
  Instant tea
Any pre-sweetened drinks:
  Hi-C
  Hawaiian Punch
  Kool-Aid (pre-sweetened)
  Carbonated soft drinks
Cereals
  Most cold cereals:
    Corn flakes
    Rice Krispies
    Bran flakes
    Alpha Bits
  All pre-sweetened cereals

  "Natural" food cereals
Baked goods (all commercial
  baked goods)
  Snack crackers (most types)
Fruits
  Canned, in corn syrup or
    sugar
  Sugared fresh fruit
  Frozen fruit in syrup
Vegetables (most canned
  vegetables)
  Candied potatoes
  Creamed vegetables
  Instant potato flakes
Meats
  Hot dogs
  Ham (cured in syrup or
    sugar)
  Pork sausage
  Italian susage
  Breakfast sausage

Frozen prepared meats:
  On-Cor Beef
  Banquet Fried Chicken
  Bacon
Snacks
  Candy
  Ice cream
  Sherbet
  Cookies
  Snack crackers
  Nuts coated with salt and
    sugar (as served in taverns
    or with beer)
Dairy products
  Processed cheese
  Margarines
  Ice Cream
  Fudgicles
  Chip dips
  Flavored cottage cheese
  Yogurt with fruit
  Frozen milk shakes
  Commercial cheese sauces
Miscellaneous
  Most liquid medicine
  Chewable tablets
  Ketchup
  Most bottled salad dressings
  Canned soups
  Commercial peanut butter
  Toothpaste
  Hershey cocoa syrup

## DIET TO CHECK FOR DYE OR FOOD COLORING ALLERGY

If you want to confirm the presence of a food coloring sensitivity, try the following:

First: Only the "allowed" foods listed below are permitted for a full week or two. Notice if the patient is better in any way. If the patient has tried this diet for two weeks and is not better, it is doubtful that dyes are the problem. If much improvement occurs in less than a week, see below.

Second: If the patient seems to improve in any way after eating only the allowed foods for one to two weeks, try a large number of the forbidden foods. Does the patient seem worse in any way? In particular, notice activity, disposition and behavior. If the patient seems worse on one occasion, try Alka-Seltzer (Gold) to see if it relieves symptoms. At this point, check with your physician for advice.

When you re-add food colors, be sure to provide as many reds, blues, greens, yellows and oranges as possible. There are many food dye colors and only one may be a problem for some people. If the right one is not consumed, you may notice no effect. After the diet, if the patient eats many colored items for three days and remains fine, dyes are probably not a problem.

### ALLOWED

Cereals
Any natural type without any food coloring

Baked goods
Any homemade types
Commercial baked goods, *if* labeled dye-free

Meats
Most are all right except those listed under "Meats" in the "Not Allowed" section on pp. 320–321.

Fish
All except those listed under "Fish" in the "Not Allowed" section on p. 320.

Vegetables (all fresh vegetables)

Fruits (all fresh fruits)

Desserts
Homemade ice cream, pudding or any item without any food coloring
Homemade candy

Beverages (any labeled without food coloring)
Grapefruit juice
Pineapple juice
Pear nectar
Guava nectar
Milk
Soybean milk

Coffee
Tea, if not colored
Homemade lemon or limeade
   from fresh fruit
Some apple cider
Some orange juice
7 Up
Colorless cream soda

Miscellaneous
  Some tub butter
  Some cheeses (white and
   specifically labeled)
  Swiss cheese
  Distilled white vinegar
  Honey
  Jam and jelly without food
   coloring (homemade)
  Homemade mayonnaise

Drugs (if a colorless liquid or
  tablet or white pill without
  any color inside or outside)

Antihistamines
  Liquid: Tacaryl Ryna
  Tablet: Actifed, Tavist,
   Fedahist
   Optimine

Asthma Drugs
  Liquids: Marax DF
   Elixicon Susp.
   Slophyllin GG
   Accurbron
   Theospan
   Aquaphyllin

  Tablets or capsules:
   Bricanyl
   Metaprel
   Somophyllin
   Chewable Theophyl
   Theophyl 225
   Slo-Phyllin 200
   Slo-Phyllin GG

## NOT ALLOWED

Cereals (any colored type)

Baked goods
  Most whole-wheat breads
  Any colored baked goods

Meats
  Luncheon meats
  Bologna
  Salami
  Kosher wieners
  Some sausage
  Some ham
  Some hamburger

Fish
  Frozen fish
  Dyed filets or sticks

Vegetables (fresh frozen may
  be dyed and not labeled
accordingly. Avoid canned,
if artificial color is listed on
label)

Fruits (any frozen or canned
fruits, if artificial color is
listed on label)

Desserts (avoid gelatins,
puddings, any box mixes,
yogurt, sherbet, ice cream or
candy unless label specifies
no food coloring)

Beverages
  Kool-Aid
  Colored pop or soda
  Some frozen juices
  All instant breakfast drinks
  All powdered beverages
  Coffee Rich (yellow dye)

Some tea mixes
Chocolate drinks or mixes
Miscellaneous
  Most butter or margarines
  Mustard
  Soy sauce
  Some vinegar
  Ketchup
  Chili or barbecue sauce
  Some cholcolate syrups
  Most cheeses

Drugs (any which are colored
  in some way)
  Cough drops
  Throat lozenges
  Most toothpaste or
    mouthwash
  Colored fluoride treatment
  Colored dental cleaner

## DIET TO CHECK FOR SOY ALLERGY

| Allowed | Not Allowed | Not Sure |
|---|---|---|
| **BEVERAGES** | | |
| Tea | see dairy products | Instant coffees |
| Coffee (brewed) | | Some hot cocoa |
| Soft drinks | | Wyler's instant bouillon |
| Fruit drinks | | |
| **BREADS** | | |
| Pepperidge Farm sandwich packets | Most biscuit, bread and muffin mixes including ready to bake types in dairy case | Lender's frozen bagels |
| Bau's English muffins | | Fresh Horizons bread |
| | Most commercial breads (all brands), rolls and English Muffins | Al Cohen's Rye |
| | Progresso Bread Crumbs | Kaufman's Rye |
| | Kellogg's Croutettes Stuffing | Kellogg's Corn Flake Crumbs |
| | Stove Top Stuffing Mixes | Horowitz-Margareten Stuffing Mix |
| | Arnold Great Stuff | |
| | Crackers (all types) | |
| | Pepperidge Farm Stuffing | |
| | Shake 'N Bake Coating Mixes | |
| | Oven Fry Coating Mixes | |
| | Croutons | |
| | Nabisco Cracker Meal | |
| | Nabisco Graham Cracker Crumbs | |

## GRAIN & GRAIN PRODUCTS

| | | |
|---|---|---|
| Pillsbury flour | Uncle Ben's Fast Cooking long grain and wild rice | Betty Crocker |
| Gold Medal flour | La Choy Fried Rice | Softasilk flour for cakes |
| Robin Hood flour | Rice-A-Roni Chicken flavored Rice | Rice-A-Roni Spanish Rice |
| Quaker Oats Quick Barley | Rice-A-Roni Beef flavored Rice | Rice-A-Roni Herb & Butter flavored rice |
| Minute Rice | Rice-A-Roni Fried Rice with Almonds | |
| Uncle Ben's Converted Rice | Quaker Corn Meal | |
| Success Rice (boil in bags) | | |
| Quaker grits | | |

## MACARONI

| | | |
|---|---|---|
| Macaroni, cooked (plain) | La Choy Chow Mein Noodles | Kraft Macaroni Cheese Dinner |
| | La Choy Rice Noodles | |
| Green Giant Lasagna | Betty Crocker Noodles Romanoff | Kraft Egg Noodle & Cheese Dinner |
| Stouffer's Lasagna | Kraft Egg Noodle & Chicken Dinner | Chef Boy-Ar-Dee canned Macaroni products |
| | Hamburger Helper (all varieties) | Stouffer's Macaroni |
| | Tuna Helper | Beef |
| | Franco-American canned Ravioli | Spaghetti to Go |
| | Franco-American canned Spaghetti | Howard Johnson's Macaroni & Cheese |
| | Lipton Lite Lunch | |
| | Betty Crocker Mug O' Lunch | |
| | Cup O Noodles | |
| | Progresso Macaroni & Beans | |
| | Swanson Hungry Man Macaroni & Cheese | |

| Allowed | Not Allowed | Not Sure |
|---|---|---|
| | Stouffer's Macaroni & Cheese | |
| | Morton Macaroni & Cheese | |
| | Swanson Macaroni & Beef | |

## CEREALS

| Allowed | Not Allowed | Not Sure |
|---|---|---|
| Most Hot and Cold Cereals | Nature Valley Granola Cereal | Beech-Nut Oatmeal Cereal |
| | Nature Valley Granola Bars | Beech-Nut Mixed Cereal |
| | Crunchola Breakfast Bars | Beech-Nut Rice Cereal |
| | Carnation Breakfast Bars | Gerber Oatmeal Cereal |
| | General Mills Breakfast Squares | |
| | Post Fortified Oat Flakes | |
| | Kellogg's Froot Loops | |
| | Kellogg's Raisin Bran | |
| | Beech-Nut Cere-meal (baby cereal) | |
| | Gerber Mixed Cereal | |
| | Gerber Rice Cereal | |
| | Gerber High Protein Cereal | |

## PASTRIES, CAKES, COOKIES, PANCAKES AND WAFFLES

| Allowed | Not Allowed | Not Sure |
|---|---|---|
| | All Betty Crocker, Jiffy, Duncan Hines, Pillsbury Cake mixes | Sara Lee Frozen donuts |
| | Jell-O Instant Cheesecake | |

All Nestlé, Quaker Oats, Betty Crocker and Duncan Hines cookie mixes
Johnston's Ready Crust
All Jiffy, Betty Crocker Pie Crust mixes
All Betty Crocker and Duncan Hines Brownie mixes
Kellogg's Pop Tarts
Mrs. Smith's frozen Pies
Morton frozen Mini Pies
All Ready to Spread Canned Frosting
Most Frosting Mixes
All Dairy case Ready to Bake Pastries
All Frozen Cakes and pastries
HoHo Fruit Pies & Cup Cakes
Most Commercially baked Cookies
Gerber Arrowroot Cookies for Toddlers
Gerber Teething Biscuits
Aunt Jemima Instant Pancakes
Pillsbury Instant Pancakes
Most Frozen Donuts

Betty Crocker Fluffy white Frosting Mix
Canned Fruit Pie Filling
Log Cabin Instant Pancakes

**PIZZA**

Appian Way Mix for *Cheese* Pizza

Appian Way mix for Regular Pizza
Stouffer's, Tony's Frozen Pizza
Chef-Boy-Ar-Dee Mix for Cheese Pizza

La Pizzeria Frozen Pizza
La Crosta Pizza Crust Mix
Robin Hood Pizza Crust Mix

## CONDIMENTS, DRESSINGS, SAUCES, SYRUPS, ETC.

| Allowed | Not Allowed | Not Sure |
|---|---|---|
| Maple Syrup | Nestlé Choco Bake, pre-melted unsweetened Chocolate | Baker's Angel Flake Coconut |
| Baker's Unsweetened Chocolate | Hershey's Semi-Sweet Chocolate chips | Hunt's Canned Tomato Sauce |
| Canned Tomato Paste | Hershey's Mini Chips | Hunt's Manwich Sauce |
| Hunt's Prima Salsa | Nestlé Semi-Sweet Chocolate Morsels | Kraft Tartar Sauce |
| Ragu Joe | Reese's Peanut Butter Chips | Good Seasons Salad Mixes |
| Progresso White Clam Spaghetti Sauce | Carnation Non-Dairy Creamer | Pfeiffer Sweet & Sour bottled Dressing |
| Hellmann's Tartar Sauce | Betty Crocker, French's Imitation Bacon bits | A1 Steak Sauce |
| Ketchup | Most Ragu Sauces | Gulden's Mustard |
| Chili Sauce | Heinz Chili Fixins | Skippy Peanut Butter |
| Del Monte Barbecue Sauce | Progresso Red Clam Spaghetti Sauce | Jif Peanut Butter |
| Most Mustard | Crockery Fixins | McCormick's Instant Seasonings & Gravies |
| Pickles | Hellmann's Kraft, Miracle Whip Mayonnaise | French's Instant Seasonings & Gravies |
| Old Fashioned Red Wing Peanut Butter | Most Bottled Salad Dressings | |
| | Kraft & Heinz Barbecue Sauces | |
| | Horseradish Sauce | |
| | Hellmann's Burger Sauce | |
| | Worcestershire Sauce | |
| | Peter Pan Peanut Butter | |

## DAIRY PRODUCTS

Butter
Cheese
Cream (real)
Eggs
Milk (cow's)
Yogurt
Milkman Hot Cocoa Mix
Swiss Miss Cocoa Mix
Evaporated Milk
Sweetened Condensed Milk

Ovaltine
Carnation Hot Cocoa Mix
Hershey's Hot Cocoa Mix

Nestlé's Quik
Alba 66
Nestlé Regular Hot Cocoa Mix

## DESSERTS, SWEETS

Jams, Jellies
Molasses
Honey
Sugar
Del Monte Mixed Fruit Cup
Jell-O Tapioca Pudding Americana
Gelatin Desserts
Birds Eye Frozen Strawberries

All Fresh Fruit
Beech-Nut Apple Betty
Beech-Nut Peach Melba
Beech-Nut Chocolate Custard

Del Monte Pudding Cups
Royal Instant Pudding
Most Jell-O Instant Pudding
Dream Whip (envelopes)
Rich's Frozen Coffee Rich

Candy
Jell-O Banana Cream pudding
Milk Chocolate Pudding (Jell-O)
Jell-O Rice Pudding

## Allowed

Beech-Nut Canned fruits
Gerber Vanilla Custard
Gerber Canned Fruits

FISH & SEAFOODS
Flounder, fresh
Haddock, fresh
Lobster, fresh
Perch, fresh
Scallops
Shrimp
Stouffer's Lobster Newburg
Gorton's of Gloucester Fish Sticks

FRUITS & JUICES
all

MEATS, POULTRY
Beef
Chicken
Lamb
Pork
Rabbit
Turkey
Veal

## Not Allowed

Stouffer's Tuna Noodle Casserole
(frozen)
Stouffer's Scallops & Shrimp Mariner
Mrs. Paul's Fish Sticks
Mrs. Paul's Fish Fillets
Van de Kamp's Fish Fillets
Most Canned Tuna packed in Oil
La Choy Shrimp Chow Mein

Green Giant Frozen Chicken Chow
   Mein
Beef Stew
Stouffer's Creamed Chicken (frozen)
Stouffer's Frozen Chicken Chow Mein
La Choy Chicken Chow Mein
La Choy Beef Pepper Oriental

## Not Sure

Chicken of the Sea Canned Tuna
   packed in Water (Vegetable broth)
Chicken of the Sea Canned Tuna
   packed in Oil
Star-Kist Canned Tuna packed in
   Water
Breast O' Chicken Canned Tuna
   packed in Water

Green Giant Salisbury Steaks
Stouffer's Frozen Chicken a la King
Stouffer's Frozen Chili
Swanson Chicken Pie
Morton Beef Pie
Swanson Beef Pie
Swanson Western Style Dinner

Stouffer's Frozen Chicken Divan
Armour Chili with Beans
Hormel Chili—No Beans
Most Cold cuts, Sausage and
Luncheon meats

La Choy Beef Chow Mein
Morton Turkey Pie
Morton Chicken Pie
Morton Steak House Beef Steak Platter
Morton Beef Dinner
Morton Turkey Dinner
Morton Chicken Dinner
Swanson Hungry Man
   Turkey Dinner
   Boneless Chicken Dinner
   Beans & Franks Dinner
   Fried Chicken
   Meatloaf
   Salisbury Steak Dinner
Weaver White Meat Chicken Roll
La Choy Meatless Chow Mein

Underwood Deviled Ham
Underwood Deviled Chicken
   (hydrolyzed vegetable protein)
Underwood Deviled Beef
Campbell's Pork & Beans

## OILS, FATS AND SHORTENINGS
Mrs. Filbert's 100% Corn Oil
   Margarine
Fleischmann's 100% Corn Oil
   Margarine
Mazola No Stick Spray
Safflower Oil
Mazola Corn Oil

Mrs. Filbert's Soft Margarine
Land O'Lakes Margarine
Imperial Margarine
Parkay Margarine
Promise Margarine
Farmdale Margarine
Blue Bonnet Margarine

| Allowed | Not Allowed | Not Sure |
|---|---|---|
| | Mazola Margarine | |
| | Pam Spray | |
| | Crisco Oil | |
| | Puritan Oil | |
| | Crisco Shortening (canned) | |

**SOUPS**

| Allowed | Not Allowed | Not Sure |
|---|---|---|
| Campbell's Onion | Progresso Canned Soups | Campbell's Vegetable Beef |
| Campbell's Scotch Broth | Campbell's Cream of Asparagus | Campbell's Beefy Mushroom |
| Campbell's Chicken Vegetable | Campbell's Manhattan Clam Chowder | Campbell's Minestrone |
| Campbell's Chili Beef | Campbell's New England Clam Chowder | Campbell's Manhandler's Beef |
| Campbell's Turkey Vegetable | Campbell's Noodles & Chicken Broth | Campbell's Chunky Beef with Vegetables |
| Campbell's Cream of Chicken | Campbell's Golden Mushroom | Campbell's Chunky Split Pea With Bacon |
| Campbell's split pea with bacon | Campbell's Green Pea | Campbell's Chunky Steak & Potato |
| Campbell's Manhandler's bean with bacon | Campbell's Old Fashioned Tomato | Wyler's Instant Chicken Bouillon |
| Campbell's Manhandler's chicken noodle | Campbell's Vegetarian Vegetable | Lipton Cup-a-Soup Chicken Noodle |
| Swift Homemade Soup Starters | Campbell's Tomato Rice | Lipton Cup-a-Soup Chicken Vegetable |
| | Campbell's Cream of Potato | |
| | Campbell's Cream of Celery | |
| | Lipton Cup-a-Soup Spring Vegetable | |
| | Lipton Cup-a-Soup Tomato | |
| | Lipton Cup-a-Soup Green Pea | |
| | Lipton Cup-a-Soup Cream of Vegetable | |
| | Lipton Cup-a-Soup Ring Noodle | |

All Fresh Vegetables
Most Canned Vegetables
Most Frozen Vegetables without Sauces
Green Giant Stuffed Green Peppers (frozen)
Green Giant Stuffed Cabbage Rolls (frozen)
Stouffer's Potatoes au Gratin (frozen)
Horowitz-Margareten Potato Pancake Mix
La Choy Chop Suey Vegetables
Green Giant Three Bean Salad
Beech-Nut Creamed Spinach (for babies)

McCain Frozen French Fries
Ore-Ida Frozen French Fries
Mrs. Paul's Fried Onion Rings (frozen)
Birds Eye frozen San Francisco Style Vegetables
Birds Eye frozen Cauliflower in Cheese Sauce
Green Giant frozen Japanese Vegetables
Green Giant frozen Chinese Vegetables
Betty Crocker Scalloped potato mix
Betty Crocker Au Gratin potato mix

Stouffer's frozen Stuffed Green Peppers
Birds Eye frozen Wisconsin Country Style Vegetables
Birds Eye frozen Chinese Stir fry vegetables
Birds Eye frozen Hawaiian vegetables
Birds Eye frozen Japanese vegetables
Green Giant frozen Hawaiian vegetables
Read Canned German Potato Salad
Grandma Brown Baked Beans
Bush's Baked Beans
B & M Baked Beans
Del Monte Cream Style Corn
Del Monte Canned Zucchini
French's potato pancake mix
French's Scalloped potato mix
French's mashed potato mix
Betty Crocker Hash Brown potato mix
Betty Crocker Potato buds
Pillsbury Hungry Jack Mashed potato mix
Martha White Old Fashioned Idaho Spud Flakes

# Appendix VII

Some medical problems are associated with specific foods. There are many exceptions, but the following symptoms have been caused by certain foods in some patients.

| Allergic-Tension Fatigue Syndrome | Aphthous Ulcers—Canker Sores | Asthma | Arthritis |
|---|---|---|---|
| Artificial coloring, preservatives, sugar (cane or beet), milk, corn, cocoa, wheat, eggs, oranges, apples, grapes, peanuts, tomatoes, food additives, artificial flavorings. Dust, mold spores and pollen. Odors from perfume or chemicals. | Citrus, pickles, apples, coffee, chocolate, potatoes, nuts and cinnamon. | Milk, eggs, wheat, or any grain, fish or shellfish, peanuts, cocoa, corn, nuts, wheat, onion, garlic. Aspirin, tartrazine dyes. | Pork (bacon, ham), lard, milk, chicken, chocolate, wheat, beef, coffee, eggs and artificial food coloring, corn, fish, turkey, lamb, spinach, cinnamon (meats seem to be a special problem). |

| Colitis | Eczema | Fluid Retention | Gall Bladder Disease |
|---|---|---|---|
| Milk, wheat, eggs, corn, cocoa, nuts, orange, pork, beef, chicken, peanut, sugar. | Milk, chocolate, nuts, peanuts, egg, mold spores, yeast, dust and pollen. | Pork | Eggs, pork, onion, chicken, milk, coffee, oranges, corn, beans, nuts. |

| Bladder Problems Enuresis | Headache | Hives | Nephrosis |
|---|---|---|---|
| Milk, eggs, citrus, corn, wheat, pork, tomato, chicken, cola, cocoa, onion, fish, cinnamon, apple, peanuts, preservatives and artificial colors. Oranges are the most common food causing adult cystitis. Molds. | Milk, chocolate, chicken, coffee, egg, corn, peanut, peas, beans, cinnamon, pork, garlic, food coloring, pollen, mold spores, dust, pets, air pollution, auto exhaust, tobacco smoke, paint fumes, perfumes, chemical odors and natural gas, wheat, orange, tea, yeast, mushrooms, peas, cane sugar, birth control pills. | Chocolate, milk, eggs, peanuts, cinnamon, preservatives, and artificial coloring or flavoring. Seasonal strawberries, melons or tomato. Aspirin, penicillin, other antibiotics. | Milk, wheat. |

| Otitis (Ear) | Nose allergies | Seizures | Blood Vessel Disease |
|---|---|---|---|
| Milk, eggs, chocolate, peanut, corn, chicken, wheat. Dust, pets, molds. | Milk, orange, corn, chocolate, wheat, artificial food coloring, egg. | Milk, yeast (vitamin B), chicken or any other food. | Chocolate, corn, nut, pork, peanuts, coffee, milk, wheat, rice, beef, shrimp, seafood, chicken, apples, peanut butter. Chemical odors, such as natural gas fumes, gasoline fumes, chlorine, air pollution, auto exhaust, soft plastic, cleaning chemicals (Lysol-phenol), perfume, polyurethane, tobacco smoke, polyester fabrics, fiberglass. Naugahyde, nap carpeting, formaldehyde, pesticides, pest strips and foam rubber. |

# Afterword

For about 50 years the practice of allergy has remained essentially the same. Diet and home changes were stressed in the early years, injection therapy and drugs later on. Allergists agree that some patients with classical allergic symptoms respond *only* to drug therapy because the cause of their medical problems is not known. There is agreement that dust, pets, pollens, molds, and so forth, can cause allergy in other patients and the recognition of sudden symptoms after the ingestion of offending foods is also acknowledged. However, only a minority of allergists believe that many patients have significant food-related allergy.

Allergists agree that the lungs, eyes, nose, skin and intestines can be altered by exposure to allergens but disagree that the bladder, muscles, joints, blood vessels, heart, kidneys and nervous system could be affected. Many allergists do not believe that chemicals such as auto exhaust, gas fumes, phenol, plastic, synthetic carpets, insecticides, preservatives, food additives and tobacco could be the cause of allergic symptoms.

A growing group of physicians called clinical ecologists now practices an expanded form of allergy. They believe that pollution and contamination of our air, food, water, soil and homes can affect our health in an adverse manner. They believe that the ingestion or odor of these items can cause acute and chronic illness, especially when these exposures are combined with stress or hormonal imbalance.

Until the medical aspects of these exposures can be approached on a national basis, avoidance of the offending items and diet appear to be a practical approach. If the latter is not practical or possible, food therapy can be administered sublingually (under the tongue) or by self-injection. This often enables patients to ingest an offending food in moderation without having symptoms. With these measures, patients often improve in days to weeks, without the need for drug therapy.

Although this form of therapy is controversial at present, an increasing number of allergy and other specialists are adopting these newer methods as more and more confirmatory scientific studies are being reported and published. It is possible that this new, non-drug-oriented approach to the practice of medicine will reveal new therapeutic methods to effectively treat some unsuspected chemical- or food-related, chronic illnesses. We must restore the natural recuperative powers within the body by reducing internal and external offending substances so that ill people no longer have to "learn to live with" their disease.

Blume, Kathleen A. 1968. *Air Pollution in the Schools and Its Effect on Our Children*. Chicago: Human Ecology Research Foundation.

Breneman, J. C. 1978. *Basics of Food Allergy*. Springfield, Illinois: Charles C. Thomas.

Coca, Arthur F. 1977. *The Pulse Test*. New York: Arco Publishing Co., Inc.

Crook, William G. 1973. *Can Your Child Read? Is He Hyperactive?* Jackson, Tennessee: Professional Books.

Crook, William G. 1978. *Are You Allergic?* Jackson, Tennessee: Professional Books (updated version of *Your Allergic Child*).

Dickey, L. D. 1976. *Clinical Ecology*. Springfield, Illinois: Charles C. Thomas.

*Forman, Robert. 1979. *How to Control Your Allergies*. New York: Larchmont Books.

*Frazier, Claude A. 1974. *Coping with Food Allergy*. New York: Quadrangle/The New York Times Book Co.

Gerrard, John W. 1973. *Understanding Allergies*. Springfield, Illinois: Charles C. Thomas.

*Golos, Natalie and Golbitz, Frances. 1979. *Coping with Your Allergies*. New York: Simon and Schuster.

Hippchen, Leonard J. 1978. *The Ecologic-Biochemical Approaches to Treatment of Delinquents and Criminals*. New York: Van Nostrand Reinhold Co.

*Hunter, Beatrice Trum. 1972. *The Fact Book on Food Additives and Your Health*. New Canaan, Connecticut: Keats Publishing Co.

*Ludeman, Kay, and Henderson, Louis. 1978. *Do It Yourself Allergy Analysis Handbook*. New Canaan, Connecticut: Keats Publishing Co.

Mackarness, Richard. 1976. *Not All in the Mind*. London and Sydney: Pan Original Books.

*Maclennan, John. 1977. *Common Sense for the Sensitive*. Hamilton, Ontario: Human Ecology Foundation of Canada.

*Mandell, Marshall. 1979. *Dr. Mandell's 5-Day Allergy Relief System*. New York: Thomas Y. Crowell.

McGee, Charles T. 1979. *How To Survive Modern Technology*. Alamo, California: Ecology Press.

McGovern, Joseph. 1980. *Nutritional Analysis System—A Physician's Manual*. San Francisco, California: Nutritional Research Publication Company.

Miller, Joseph B. 1972. *Food Allergy: Provocative Testing and Injection Therapy*. Springfield, Illinois: Charles C. Thomas.

*Oski, Frank. 1977. *Don't Drink Your Milk*. New York: Wyden Books.

Ott, John. 1976. *Health and Light*. New York: Pocket Books.

Pfeiffer, Guy O. and Nikel, Casimir M. 1980. *The Household Environment and Chronic Illness*. Springfield, Illinois: Charles C. Thomas.

Randolph, Theron G. 1972. *Human Ecology and Susceptibility to the Chemical Environment*. Springfield, Illinois: Charles C. Thomas.

Randolph, Theron, G. and Moss, Ralph W. 1980. *An Alternative Approach to Allergies*. New York: Harper and Row.

*Rapp, Doris J. 1979. *Allergies and the Hyperactive Child*. New York: Sovereign Books; Simon and Schuster. (Cornerstone softcover).

Rinkle, H., Randolph, T., and Zeller, M. 1951. *Food Allergy*. Norwalk, Connecticut: New England Foundation of Allergic and Environmental Diseases.

*Rowe, Albert, and Rowe, Jr., Albert. 1972. *Food Allergy*. Springfield, Illinois: Charles C. Thomas.

Schauss, Alexander, 1980. *Diet, Crime and Delinquency*. Berkeley, California: Parkerhouse.

Speer, F. 1970. *Allergy of the Nervous System*. Springfield, Illinois: Charles C. Thomas.

Thomas, L. 1979. Caring and Cooking for the Allergic Child. New York: Sterling.

Trites, Ronald W., Tryphonas, H., and Ferguson, B. 1978. Treatment of hyperactivity in a child with allergies to food. In *Case Studies in Hyperactivity*, ed. Marvin J. Fine. Springfield, Illinois: Charles C. Thomas.

von Hilsheimer, George. 1970. *How to Live with Your Special Child*. Washington, D.C.: Acropolis.

von Hilsheimer, George. 1974. *Allergy, Toxins, and the Learning Disabled Child*. San Rafael, California: Academic Therapy Publications.

Wunderlich, Ray C. 1973. *Allergy, Brains and Children Coping*. St. Petersburg, Florida: Johnny Reads, Inc.

*Books have foods and cooking sections.

# *Index*